Safety Guide for Health Care Institutions

Fourth Edition

By Linda F. Chaff

AHA®
American Hospital Publishing, Inc.,
a wholly owned subsidiary of the
American Hospital Association

National Safety Council

Library of Congress Cataloging-in-Publication Data

Chaff, Linda F.
Safety guide for health care institutions. — 4th ed. / by Linda F. Chaff.
p. cm.
Includes bibliographical references.
ISBN 1-55648-038-5
1. Hospitals—Safety measures. I. Title.
RA969.9.C43 1989 89-37764
362.1'1'0684—dc20 CIP

Catalog no. 181148

Printed in the U.S.A.

AHA is a service mark of the American Hospital Association used under license by American Hospital Publishing, Inc.

Text set in Bookman Light
4M—10/89—0245

Audrey Kaufman, Project Editor
Linda Conheady, Manuscript Editor
Sophie Yarborough, Editorial Assistant
Marcia Bottoms, Managing Editor
Peggy DuMais, Production Coordinator
Marcia Vecchione, Designer
Brian Schenk, Book Division Director

Contents

About the Author

Linda F. Chaff is president of Chaff & Co. (Clarendon Hills, Illinois), an organization that develops management systems for health care organizations and corporations. She has more than 13 years' experience in safety program development and training, and she has written articles in professional journals and books on motivation, leadership skills, safety, security, training, and management concepts. She recently wrote and self-published a manual entitled *Progressive Waste Management: A Policy Guide for Healthcare.*

Previously, Ms. Chaff was director of Protection Services at Monongalia General Hospital in Morgantown, West Virginia, where she developed, implemented, and evaluated a comprehensive loss-prevention management program that minimized loss by targeting its causes—such as fire destruction, accidents, medical malpractice claims, and patient/employee complaints. She is past chair of the National Safety Council's Health Care Section, is a member of the National Safety Council's International Advisory Committee on Safety and Health, and is on the Advisory Board for Rusting Publication's Nursing Home Security and Safety Management newsletter.

List of Figures

List of Tables

Preface

Health care facilities operate in a unique environment. No other business brings together such a diversity of services, people, and equipment. Unlike other services, providing medical care demands human performance with no margin for error, 365 days a year, 24 hours a day, with no downtime, holidays, or lapses in service.

Health care institutions are entrusted with the safety of several distinct groups—employees, visitors, volunteers, and, increasingly, members of the community—as well as the life and health of their patients. In many cases, particularly in long-term care or psychiatric facilities, patients are unable to care for themselves or ensure their own safety. As a result, unsafe acts, equipment failures, and other dangerous conditions in these institutions may have especially serious—even tragic—consequences. This unique environment makes safety a high priority.

Compounding the risks inherent in the operation of health care organizations are rapid and dramatic shifts in society and technology. The past 10 years have seen numerous changes unprecedented in their effect on health care. Acquired immunodeficiency syndrome (AIDS), for example, poses formidable dilemmas both for society and for medical facilities. Health care institutions must care for AIDS patients compassionately and safely while ensuring employee safety. Advances in technology continue at an astounding rate, giving the industry tools, such as lasers, that can greatly enhance treatment and concurrently introduce new risks. Changing demographics influence health care as greater numbers of people become geriatric and require special care. Economic factors, resulting from lower occupancy rates and large health care chains, continue to tighten competition in the health care market. Negative publicity from unsafe conditions can easily damage a facility's competitive position; safe conditions can enhance patient care and attract new patients.

Regulations affecting health care continue to multiply. As facilities produce more hazardous waste and use more chemicals with treatment benefits but potential side effects, regulatory control expands, adding to the basic safety requirements. Medical institutions must fulfill the requirements of both government and voluntary agencies, and they must keep up with rapid changes in standards.

Finally, there are health care's rapidly increasing liability costs. In the past, patients were reluctant to sue their neighborhood hospital or doctor, but now, with larger, less personal facilities and health care corporations, litigation is often the choice for patients who feel that their treatment was inadequate, negligent, or deleterious.

Clearly, a comprehensive response is required. The health care institution must adopt the attitude that mounting losses can be averted. A well-planned, all-inclusive safety program with the commitment and participation of the entire staff can stem the tide of escalating risks. The benefits of such a program are many: Accidents can be reduced, along with workers' compensation claims and lost work time. Citations and penalties from regulatory agencies can be avoided through compliance with regulations. Compliance with these regulations will assist in gaining accreditation from the Joint Commission on Accreditation of Healthcare Organizations. Liability for accidents and injuries that occur on facility premises will decrease as the facility is made a safer place in which to work, stay, or visit. The staff will be better prepared for emergencies (such as fire or other disaster), limiting the potential for damage to life, health, and property. By encouraging all staff members to participate, a feeling of teamwork can be established that boosts employee morale and productivity.

These advantages represent just a few of the benefits that effective safety management can provide under the right conditions. This manual outlines a comprehensive program for achieving these goals as well as specific objectives for an individual facility. Chapter 1 provides guidelines for planning the safety program and describes four preparatory steps—obtaining administration support, conducting the needs assessment, setting priorities, and developing policies and procedures. Chapter 2 provides essential information on regulatory and voluntary compliance agencies affecting health care. The various components of the overall safety program—the safety committee, departmental safety, patient safety, fire safety, emergency preparedness, and hazardous and infectious materials management—are described in chapters 3 through 8. Chapter 9 provides practical advice for implementing an incident reporting system, and chapter 10 is devoted to training, a part of safety that is essential and often overlooked. Chapter 11 focuses on the unique needs of mental health facilities as they face growing safety requirements and expanded liability. Finally, the key to success of any safety program is ongoing evaluation. Chapter 12 identifies the problems encountered during the evaluation phase and provides some solutions.

No health care organization can afford to operate without a strong, comprehensive safety program. This text provides the framework and the resources from which a comprehensive safety program can be built and tailored to the facility's unique needs.

Acknowledgments

With heartfelt gratitude, I thank the many people whose advice, ideas, and expertise not only made possible but greatly enhanced the development of this book:

Foremost among all contributors is Cindy Blevins-Doll, whose agility and acuity in writing and researching, as well as her flexibility in adjusting to the demands of a rigorous schedule, have been invaluable. Cindy's perseverance coupled with her creativity made work on this project enjoyable and exciting.

As primary technical editor, Joe McFadden, safety director of Rose Medical Center, provided his knowledge and technical skill in the development stages of the manuscript. I am indebted to Joe for his diligence in providing thorough critique and feedback.

Mike Peltier, section administrator of the National Safety Council's Health Care Section, provided his skills as primary reviewer and greatly facilitated the initial stages of manuscript development.

I am grateful to Audrey Kaufman, product line manager, American Hospital Publishing, Inc., for her fine job of editing and offering critical suggestions and recommendations.

Roberta Carroll, Ron Cundiff, Carol J. Doyle, Lawrence P. Gallagher, Linda Glasson, Merrie Healy, Ed Mendenhall, and Ed Savard contributed in practical and incisive ways. I appreciate their expert input and their willingness to share ideas and provide insights along the way.

My thanks to Marilyn Benedict, chair, and members of the Health Care Section of the National Safety Council, who approved and encouraged the inception of this book and who were accessible to answer questions and offer their expertise.

The commitment and dedication of everyone involved in all aspects of this book's publication is greatly appreciated. Their patience in advising and supporting me made an otherwise insurmountable task a delight.

Chapter 1
Planning a Safety Program

A health care facility is a complex institution comprising numerous, widely diverse departments and functions. Perhaps more than any other service, providing health care means assuming multiple roles: The facility becomes a hotel, a restaurant, a retail business, a cleaning service, a laboratory, and so on. Because these roles may contrast greatly, the departments that administer these services tend to act autonomously. Each department, therefore, generates risks that may be unique to it alone. What results is a broad variety of risks that may be managed in an uncoordinated, disjointed way.

Because of the complexity of routine facility operation and the tendency of departments to act independently of one another, thorough planning and coordination are essential to a comprehensive and successful safety program. Commitment from all sectors of the facility, particularly top management, should be obtained in order to encourage interaction. A facilitywide needs assessment (also referred to as a risk assessment) must be conducted before priorities can be identified and preventive measures can be instituted, and safety guidelines in the form of written policies and procedures that are practical and understandable must be developed. These four preparatory steps—obtaining administration support, conducting the needs assessment, setting priorities, and writing policies and procedures—provide the foundation for a results-oriented safety program.

□ Administration Support

The impetus for safety must emanate from the highest echelons in the health care facility hierarchy—the board of directors and the chief executive officer (CEO). Enthusiastic support for the program from these officials not only provides the authority needed to begin planning but demonstrates to employees that the safety program is a job requirement rather than just a piece of paper. Administration backing also enhances the relationship between employees and the CEO by showing top management's concern for the safety and health of workers.

Without the administration's clear commitment, safety directors cannot generate the involvement and support of the staff. Employees can sense when safety is only being given lip service without any serious intentions to implement procedures. They react by returning the same halfhearted commitment. The end result is often a frustrated safety director, a largely ignored safety program, and escalating risks to the facility.

The board and the CEO have the ability to change this scenario. Their actions carry weight among employees, supervisors, and department heads. A good way to demonstrate administration support for the program is through a formal statement that underscores the importance of the safety program. This statement should go to all staff members and include:

- An introduction to the safety program
- The objectives of the system, including protection of employees, patients, visitors, the community, the environment, and the facility
- A statement investing authority for the program in one person or department
- Encouragement of active departmental cooperation
- Assurance that safety responsibilities will be incorporated into all job descriptions
- An explanation of the importance of safety and the administration's ongoing support
- A brief discussion of the elements of the safety system, such as fire prevention, incident reporting, and emergency preparedness

Figure 1-1 (see p. 9) shows a prototype administration support statement. It may be advisable for the administration to write two separate statements—a formal one to be given to managers that establishes responsibility and authority; and a second, less formal statement for employees that explains the safety program but emphasizes protection of employees and basic employee responsibilities. The statement for employees could be as informal as a letter, which will personalize the message.

For those health care facilities that already have a safety program in place but want to update or expand it, communicating the goals of the program is still a necessary step. Employees must understand the reasons for new requirements and changes in their jobs. In this case, the administration should emphasize the need to update procedures as new risks develop. The administration should reiterate its continuing support for a safe working environment for all involved.

Finally, the CEO should translate verbal support into monetary support. Enough funds should be budgeted for safety to cover a needs assessment, program development, personnel, equipment, training, and ongoing monitoring. The CEO should view this financial commitment as an investment in a system that will provide numerous returns in the form of reduced liability, improved employee morale, fewer accidents, and other factors that favorably influence the well-being of the facility.

☐ The Needs Assessment

After the administration has demonstrated its support through statements and other publicity and budgetary support, the next step is to get a clear picture of the current safety practices and programs within the facility. Risks can then be identified in order to determine the facility's safety needs.

Discovering existing risks and conditions is a step often neglected in the rush to begin a safety program. Many health care facility managers assume that the organization's insurance carrier will identify all exposures before writing coverage. Although information from insurance inspections can be useful, it is limited. Smaller exposures may escape notice. Factors such as employee attitude and satisfaction will not be included in the insurer's assessments.

Therefore, safety builds on, but is not limited to, insurance concerns. A safety needs assessment addresses the less tangible but equally significant elements of safety—such as employee commitment, management participation, and acceptance of the program as part of the facility's routine. The health care facility's assessment, unlike that of the insurance company, will directly involve employees—and they are the ones who have firsthand knowledge of the facility and the jobs as well as the risks in both.

Preparing for the Needs Assessment

The needs assessment is a survey of the current programs, prevailing attitudes, and risks presently affecting the operation. The assessment is conducted by a survey team. If there is a safety committee, the survey team can be chosen from the committee's members. Three to four people will usually suffice. Members should be appointed based on aptitude and enthusiasm. Preferably, the survey team will include the safety director and representatives from administration, management, and employees—this constitutes the core team. The core team should survey every department or facility area. In each department, the core team will work closely with that department manager, who, for that part of the survey, becomes a temporary member of the survey team.

Before beginning the assessment, the survey team should be trained in conducting visual inspections. This training can be as simple as a short briefing that includes a discussion of some common problems and how to detect them. With the right training, such hazards as improper storage of compressed gas cylinders and broken ladders, for example, can be easily detected. Department managers should be present; they should be instructed about their role in these departmental surveys, which is to facilitate and assist in the inspection of their departments.

Checklists are useful when conducting visual inspections. Many good resources exist for developing checklists, including the Joint Commission on Accreditation of Healthcare Organizations's (Joint Commission's) annual *Accreditation Manual for Hospitals.* A prototype safety inspection checklist has been included in appendix C of this guide. With some modifications to reflect each facility's structure, this checklist can serve as an important assessment tool.

In addition to visual inspections, a comprehensive needs assessment includes a review of all pertinent records. The records organizations keep can give the survey team a sense of the direction of the safety program, including its past accomplishments and oversights. Records to be reviewed include:

- Accident/incident reports
- Safety committee minutes
- Joint Commission survey reports
- Governmental agency inspection results (for example, those from the Occupational Safety and Health Administration (OSHA), the Environmental Protection Agency, the Nuclear Regulatory Commission, state and county health departments, and fire marshal reports)
- Insurance company inspection records

- Workers' compensation statistics
- Policies and procedures

As part of preparation for the assessment, these and other records from at least the past year should be gathered and summarized by the safety director, with the help of his or her staff or the safety committee. The information must be condensed because of its sheer bulk. It would be too time-consuming for those involved in the assessment to review, for example, every incident report from the past two years. Instead, these documents should be translated into statistics and trends, such as the percentage of back injuries, needle sticks, slips and falls, workers' compensation claims, and so forth.

Conducting the Assessment

After the aforementioned preparation has been done, the team members are ready to begin the assessment. A thorough facilitywide assessment should not be attempted in one day. The survey team should probably spend no more than an hour at a time actually conducting the assessment. The team members, of course, have other responsibilities and will begin to resent an assessment that monopolizes too much of their time. An hour in each department will provide a cursory look at the existing situation. Perhaps no more than two departments should be inspected in one day (for example, one in the morning and another in the afternoon). Primarily, the surveyors will be looking for four major elements:

- Condition of the physical facility
- Prevailing attitudes and actions
- Safety programs in place
- Condition of equipment

The Physical Facility

The first area of assessment is the safety of the physical facility. It can be determined using resources such as Joint Commission standards, OSHA regulations, fire codes, and a checklist. The safety of the facility includes not only how it was built (which little can be done about now), but also how it is being used: Are exits blocked? Have storage practices created a fire hazard? Are support structures in need of repair? Is the area secure? The survey team should consult knowledgeable resources such as maintenance and engineering personnel. Most important, survey team members should talk to the people who know the particular area of the facility best—employees who work there every day.

Attitudes and Actions

By some estimates, up to 90 percent of accidents are caused by unsafe acts (rather than by unsafe conditions). These dangerous acts can stem from a variety of causes—inadequate training, confusing directions, tiredness, carelessness, and so forth. Impractical procedures or safety measures may also contribute to unsafe behavior. For instance, an accident reporting system that requires several different lengthy reports to be filled out may discourage reporting. The survey team should observe the behavior of employees and the attitudes their actions convey: Are they rushed? Do they follow standard procedure for routine tasks? To assess attitudes and actions, interaction with employees is critical. The survey team should assure employees that they are not evaluating the employees' job performance but are looking for better ways to protect valuable workers from hazardous practices. Employees should be encouraged to make suggestions for improvement. The importance of an ongoing dialogue with employees during the assessment and throughout the safety process cannot be overemphasized.

Existing Programs and Practices

The third assessment area is an evaluation of the effectiveness of safety programs already in place. Questions to be asked might include the following:

- Is there a safety committee that meets regularly?
- Are problems investigated and resolved?
- Is there a written policy for matters such as extension cords and adapters, emergency preparedness, hazardous waste, and so forth?
- Are program requirements actually followed?
- Are there specific policies for the departments as well as policies addressing the entire facility?
- Are written procedures understandable and effective?

This is the time when many of the records will be helpful, most particularly policies and procedures, but also accident statistics, workers' compensation records, regulatory inspection reports, and the like. Policies and procedures are the written guidelines for programs and, as such, must be reviewed for clarity and effectiveness in achieving their purpose. Once again, employees' views are helpful in evaluating present programs.

Equipment

The team should determine the safety of the equipment in each department. Here, the advice of maintenance personnel becomes crucial. Basic resources, such as safety checklists and manufacturers' instructions, will also explain what to look for in equipment. The survey team should determine whether a system of preventive maintenance is in place. Is equipment regularly inspected? Is there an "alert" or recall program in operation for defective equipment? Is defective equipment repaired or discarded? Is broken equipment allowed to be used? Survey team members should keep in mind the goal of equipment management: to repair and maintain equipment *before* it causes an accident or injury.

Results of the Assessment

Completing an assessment that includes these four elements—facility, attitudes, programs, and equipment—not only provides the survey team with an in-depth look at the existing safety condition of the facility but, equally significant, it fosters a new relationship among the CEO, the managers, and the employees. Including administration on the team demonstrates—through actions—top management's commitment to the safety program. Because employees and managers are also represented, the survey team becomes a model of the teamwork vital to the success of the program. Finally, because of the constant interaction between the assessment team and the department employees, employees feel that they are included in the decision-making process. This interaction builds commitment to a program employees feel they have helped create and fosters a team effort for problem solving.

Priority Setting

The assessment will generate much useful information, but this can be lost if it is not organized and condensed. The results of the assessment—both the visual inspections and the review of records—should be summarized in writing in an assessment report. The assessment report could also indicate the conclusions to which assessment results point. For example, if records indicate a continuous increase in needle sticks among nursing or housekeeping staff, the report could propose reasons to explain the increase, such as lack of proper receptacles or a feeling among nurses of being rushed. It is important, however, not to place blame on the employees or on a specific individual. Safety problems more often suggest deficiencies in management and planning than in willful employee negligence.

The completed report should be submitted to the administration and a meeting should be called to discuss it and set priorities for program development. The survey team, representatives from the department with safety responsibilities, and the CEO are among those who should be present. The survey team should be prepared to make recommendations, but it must also remain open to the suggestions and feedback of others.

In setting priorities, there are four major factors to consider for each safety condition uncovered by the assessment:

- *Type.* What kinds of problems have been created by this particular condition: Accidents? Employee dissatisfaction? Injuries? Near-misses? Perhaps a policy or procedure is not being followed. Does this create hazards? If so, what type? In this category, it is important to remember that accidents are not the only type of problem caused by unsafe conditions. Other problems include employee resentment, unfavorable public relations, patient anxiety, and security vulnerabilities. The types of problems can be many, and all bear risks for the facility.
- *Frequency.* How often has this condition created this problem? Has it generated an ongoing risk? Does an accident occur frequently because of the condition? The frequency should be noted for every type of problem.
- *Severity.* How severe is this deficiency? Is it likely to cause major loss? Could it mean regulatory inspections and fines or Joint Commission accreditation problems? Could it attract adverse publicity, cause strikes, offend unions? Again, personnel and community reactions should be considered in determining severity. For instance, employees and the community may be alarmed at having AIDS patients in the facility even though protective measures have been implemented. The possible consequences of this fear (such as civil suits and OSHA censure) must be considered, along with ways to allay the anxiety.
- *Probability.* Decision-makers must project the likelihood of each consequence of an unsafe condition, based on past history and educated guesses about future trends. For example, is continuing economic loss likely from workers' compensation claims? Answers should be based on past records as well as projections by experts (such discussions of future trends are often found in safety journals and reference books, even newspapers).

A consideration of these factors will yield a clearer picture of how problems should be prioritized. No matter how the priorities are arranged, steps should be taken immediately to assure employees that the hazards will be corrected. A memo could be written to inform employees that the identified problems in each of their areas have not been ignored, but that more severe conditions must be treated first for the protection of employees and patients.

The prioritized results will then serve as a basis for long- and short-term goals. Having a written set of goals will help in measuring the success of the program. Achievable short-term goals will also contribute to a feeling of accomplishment when participants can see on paper the progress they are making.

□ Policy and Procedure Writing

After priorities have been identified and goals set, the next step is to write or revise policies and procedures. These policies and procedures form the heart of the program. They outline the commitment to the program, define responsibilities, and provide details for the procedures required by the program. They can also be an excellent resource for safety training. Figure 1-2 (see p. 10) shows a sample policy and procedure form.

Written policies and procedures serve as evidence of the facility's intention to provide a safe environment for employees and patients. These documents can be useful in defending the facility during litigation (of course, proof of actually carrying out the procedures is also necessary). Moreover, the Joint Commission requires policies and procedures for accreditation, as do governmental agencies such as OSHA, for certain programs such as hazard communication.

Together with the safety committee, the safety director writes and revises policies and procedures (the role of the safety committee is discussed in chapter 3). These policies must be developed for each of the major elements, such as accident prevention and reporting, hazardous and infectious waste, fire prevention, and so forth. In addition, specific procedures must be written for each policy. An infectious waste policy, for example, will include procedures for collecting, storing, and disposing of each of the different types of infectious waste.

When writing policies and procedures, the following areas should be addressed:

- *Policy.* What is the policy? A short statement should explain the policy and the reasons for it, as well as its place in the framework of the entire safety program.
- *Responsibility.* Who is responsible for ensuring that the procedures are followed? Who bears the responsibility for carrying out the procedures? These people should be referred to by title. For example, "The infection control nurse has the primary responsibility for coordinating the bloodborne infectious disease protection program."
- *Procedures.* Specifically, what must each of the participants do? Procedures should be step-by-step instructions that can be used in training.

After policies and procedures have been written, they should be approved in writing by the CEO and the chief officer of the medical staff. They should then be reviewed at least annually for effectiveness, employee reactions, regulatory developments, and changes in operations. The policies and procedures should be consolidated into a policy and procedure manual, preferably a three-ring binder, that also includes the goals of the program and the statement of administration support. This manual can then serve as the comprehensive resource for the safety program.

Integrating Risk Management Concepts

As risks to health care facilities escalate, you may be hearing a great deal about risk management. Your facility may even have a risk management department or employ a risk manager. Whatever the circumstances, in developing a safety program it is important to integrate risk management concepts in order to deal more comprehensively with the myriad possibilities for loss in the health care setting.

Risk management refers to a philosophy that all risks can be managed through an ordered system of protection. This system includes the traditional elements of safety, such as accident prevention, emergency preparedness, and fire prevention. It also includes principles that some traditional safety programs have not included, such as liability control, employee motivation, professional development, patient relations, risk financing, and quality assurance concepts.

Effective risk management recognizes that risks involve people and so places a major emphasis on communicating with and properly relating to the facility's people—employees, managers, physicians, administrators, patients, volunteers, visitors, and members of the community. Soliciting ideas and thoughts, helping staff grow through training and development, and explaining the reasoning behind programs are all of paramount importance in risk management. Risk management is a comprehensive system owing to its holistic approach to individuals as much as to its integrated prevention programs.

In this way, successful risk management is all-inclusive. It forms a tightly woven net of protection for the facility. Consequently, in order to boost the effectiveness of safety measures, risk management concepts should be integrated into the safety program. Safety problems should be considered in relation to each other and to the operation of the entire facility. The concerns and reactions of people should be brought to bear in decision making, and teamwork should be encouraged. By integrating concepts of overall risk management into safety concepts, facilities can enhance not only the safety program but employee morale, financial stability, and patient care as well.

Conclusion

Four major preparatory steps—administration support, needs assessment, priority setting, and policy and procedure development—provide the foundation for a systemwide safety program. Although the scope of these elements may seem extensive, thorough planning is essential to the program's success. It is also important to integrate risk management concepts into the safety program, such as liability control, employee motivation, professional development, patient relations, risk financing, and quality assurance. Such a comprehensive, well-planned program can become a dynamic force in maintaining the safety of the institution for years to come.

Figure 1-1. Prototype Administration Support Statement

(Name of facility)'s policy is to do all that is reasonable to prevent injury to persons and damage to property and to protect the employees, the facility, the patients (residents), the environment, and the public from injury, fire, or other damage. In order to achieve these goals, (name of facility) is instituting a comprehensive safety program. The program will be a well-planned and thoroughly organized approach to ensuring safety.

The administration urges the active cooperation and commitment of all departments and employees. In implementing the program, safety responsibilities shall become incorporated into all job descriptions, and staff will be trained in fulfilling new duties. Safety will become part of job performance evaluation, and ongoing dialogue and feedback will be encouraged.

(Name of facility)'s administration supports this program in its promotion of employee safety and health. The administration also supports the policy that everything within reason shall continue to be done throughout the facility to maintain or enhance comprehensive safety.

[*Note: The following are suggested elements. These may differ, depending on the facility.*]

The safety program will include:

- Safety policies and procedures for all departments and services
- Incident reporting and investigation
- Emergency preparedness
- Hazardous materials and hazardous waste programs
- Fire protection
- Patient safety measures
- A safety committee
- Safety education and training

The primary responsibility for coordinating and supervising the safety program shall rest with the (title). (He/she) will regularly consult with and advise the administration on safety matters and is responsible for the development, implementation, and monitoring of the safety program. (He/she) will have the authority necessary to carry out program activities.

______________________ ______________________

[CEO] [Chairman, Board of Trustees]

____

[Chief Officer, Medical Staff]

Figure 1-2. Sample Policy and Procedure Form

Subject: Product Recall

Policy # 3-1 Page 1 of 1

Effective Date 4/26/89

Approved ______

Replaces # 3-1 Dated 4/13/89

Policy:

It is the policy of (facility) to take corrective action to provide for the safety and well-being of all patients, staff, and visitors whenever information concerning products or equipment purchased by this institution is thought to be dangerous or hazardous to one's health.

Responsibility:

The director of safety will take all necessary steps to ensure timely completion of recall action, and is designated product safety coordinator. It is the responsibility of the facility's product safety coordinator to receive, evaluate, and act upon all information concerning product recalls or equipment hazards. In the absence of the director, the vice-president will act as product safety coordinator.

Procedure:

A. The product safety coordinator (or authorized designee) will receive all recall notices, whether by telephone, telegraph, letter, or in person. Telephone notices are most likely to be those requiring immediate attention. Each recall notice will be immediately evaluated for priority, with Class I (urgent) recalls taking precedence over other matters, at least until it has been determined that no imminent hazard exists (for example, the facility does not have the offending product, it has been quarantined, or the defect has been corrected).
B. It shall be the responsibility of all department managers to communicate this policy to the employees under their supervision. Department managers will be responsible for reporting incidents, product recalls, and device failures promptly to the product safety coordinator.
C. Any changes or additions to this policy will be issued from the office of the president.

Chapter 2

Regulatory and Voluntary Compliance Agencies

Throughout this century, patient care has steadily and dramatically increased in effectiveness. For example, one of the leading causes of death at the turn of the century—influenza—has been reduced in most cases to a minor illness rather than a life-threatening disease. More patients than ever with critical injuries and other acute conditions survive because of advanced technology and procedures. However, the same high-tech atmosphere that saves lives also brings more risks—to hospital employees, to the community, to patients, and to the environment.

Modern miracles of technology may create electrical and fire hazards or may malfunction. Wonder drugs can have serious side effects. Substances that make treatment easier or more successful, such as anesthesia gases and radioactive materials, may pose hazards to employees and the environment. The everyday operation of a health care facility may engender numerous risks through unsafe conditions such as wet floors or blocked fire exits.

These sources of risk have resulted in increased regulation by agencies seeking to ensure that health care facilities maintain a safe environment. These organizations can be divided into two principal types—governmental and voluntary.

□ Governmental Compliance Agencies

Governmental compliance agencies are those organizations that the government—federal, state, or local—has endowed with the authority to establish regulations and enforce them. Many times, the rules these agencies promulgate have the force of law, and violators may be subject to criminal penalties. Other times, these agencies may publish guidelines rather than enforce laws, but the agencies may still base their inspections and citations on these guidelines or recommendations.

Governmental compliance agencies publish information and operate offices where concerned individuals can call for answers or assistance. As government entities, they are public servants, but all too often employers fail to make use of this resource. The employees of these agencies are often happy to help with any concerns you may have and, at the very least, will put you in contact with an organization that can assist you, if they cannot. Information on how to contact each agency is listed in this chapter.

Occupational Safety and Health Administration

In 1970, during the Nixon administration, Congress passed the Occupational Safety and Health Act, which created an agency controlled by the Department of Labor and established regulations requiring employers to ensure safe and healthful working conditions for employees in the workplace. The Occupational Safety and Health Act gave every employee the right to a reasonably secure, risk-free environment, which the employer must maintain. The agency created by this act is called the Occupational Safety and Health Administration, or OSHA.

Soon after its birth, OSHA began to develop regulations for employers that governed workplace safety. It summarized the responsibility of employers in its General Duty clause, namely that the employer must provide "employment and a place of employment which are free from recognized hazards that are causing or are likely to cause death or serious physical harm" to employees.

On the basis of this foundation, OSHA moved on to write other regulations on more specific safety issues for various industries. Once these regulations were established, it became the task of all employers and employees to familiarize themselves with those that applied to them and to comply conscientiously with these regulations at all times.

The Occupational Safety and Health Administration has issued numerous regulations that affect health care facilities, especially in the area of general safety. For example, there are OSHA rules covering the use of ladders and scaffolds, the condition of exits, electrical safety, lifting techniques, and the use of personal protective equipment. Moreover, the Joint Commission on Accreditation of Healthcare Organizations (Joint Commission) often relies partly on basic OSHA safety regulations in developing its accreditation criteria.

Other areas of OSHA regulation and guidance for health care facilities include the storage and transportation of compressed gas cylinders, the control of waste anesthetic gas, the handling of cytotoxic (antineoplastic) drugs, and the use of X-ray equipment. In addition, OSHA has published guidelines for protecting workers from occupational exposure to AIDS, hepatitis B, and other blood-borne diseases. The agency intends to promulgate a blood-borne infectious disease standard with the force of law by 1991.

Finally, although this is by no means an exhaustive list, OSHA oversees compliance with its Hazard Communication Standard. First published in 1983, this standard gives employees the "right to know" what hazardous chemicals they work with. Whereas the rule at first only applied to manufacturing industries, in 1987 OSHA expanded the standard to cover all employers, including health care facilities. Under the "right-to-know" standard, as it came to be called, all employees must be informed about the chemicals they work with—they must know the chemicals' hazards and how to protect themselves. The Hazard Communication Standard has a number of specific requirements for employers, including a written program and training for employees.

The Occupational Safety and Health Administration enforces its requirements through workplace inspections. These inspections may occur for the following reasons:

- Imminent danger
- Catastrophes or fatal accidents
- Employee complaints
- Programmed inspections for high-hazard industries
- Follow-up inspections

Inspections are conducted to determine whether safety and health hazards are being overlooked by the employer and, when necessary, citations are issued and fines levied.

If the potential harm represents immediate threat to the health or life of employees, OSHA will take immediate steps to remove the hazards. Otherwise, OSHA may issue a citation that will result in penalties or civil or criminal fines. However, OSHA assures employers that consideration is given to the appropriateness of the penalty, the severity of the violation, the size of the facility, the good faith of the employer, and the record of previous violations.

Many resources exist to help the staff and supervisors of health care facilities understand what OSHA expects of them. This awareness is intrinsic to an effective safety program, because OSHA was established to ensure workplace safety. In many ways, OSHA standards and guidelines relate directly to the health care facility. Understanding them can greatly enhance safety and the smooth operation of the facility. For more information, contact your OSHA regional office (see table 2-1 on p. 22) or call or write to the federal office.

Occupational Safety and Health Administration, Frances Perkins Building, 200 Constitution Avenue, Washington, DC 20210, 202/523-6091.

U.S. Environmental Protection Agency

The Environmental Protection Agency (EPA) exercises control over the release of harmful materials into the environment and, like OSHA, has written both legislation and guidance. These rules and recommendations define which substances can be hazardous to human health and the environment, outline formalized procedures for handling these materials, govern the operation of waste disposal sites, and establish a system for dealing with environmental accidents such as leaks or spills.

As patient care becomes more and more complex, health care facilities must frequently deal with hazardous chemicals during routine operation. Whereas OSHA's Hazard Communication Standard covers the use of these substances by employees in the performance of their jobs, EPA rules apply primarily to the effects of the materials on the environment. The Environmental Protection Agency's purview extends to infectious wastes because of their potential danger to humans and the environment, although the degree of possible harm remains a matter of debate. In order to effect a comprehensive system of control for dangerous wastes, the EPA has published numerous rules and guidelines. The following have the greatest effect on health care:

- *Clean Air Act.* In 1970, Congress passed this act to empower the EPA to set permissible levels for the emission of hazardous substances into the air. Congress is currently considering changes and reauthorization regarding this act.
- *Clean Water Act.* In an effort to buttress the 1972 Federal Water Pollution Control Act, the Clean Water Act was passed in 1977. This act limits the discharge of hazardous substances into our waterways. The act estab-

lished the National Pollutant Discharge Elimination System (NPDES), which requires permits for the discharge of harmful materials into water. In 1987, this act was bolstered by a congressional reauthorization.

- *Toxic Substances Control Act (TSCA) of 1976.* This legislation regulates the manufacture, distribution, and use of toxic chemicals. It requires manufacturers to notify the EPA when proposing new chemicals, and it provides for the regular assessment of existing hazardous chemicals. The Toxic Substances Control Act may limit or prohibit the use of some chemicals, and this may have an impact on health care. For example, the use of polychlorinated biphenyls (PCBs), except in a totally enclosed system, has been disallowed. The transformers and capacitors in some older facilities may contain PCBs and may not always be regarded as a totally enclosed system.
- *The Resource Conservation and Recovery Act (RCRA) of 1976.* This is the act of most interest to health care facilities and other waste generators. It establishes a system for the control of hazardous wastes from the time they are generated until their final disposal, from "cradle to grave." The act divides waste generators into categories based on the amount of waste generated; requires permits for generators, transporters, and disposal facilities; and sets up a system whereby wastes are tracked from generation to disposal. Chapter 6 discusses RCRA's health care facility requirements in greater detail.
- *Comprehensive Environmental Response, Compensation, and Liability Act (CERCLA) of 1980.* Called "Superfund," this act allocates funding and direction for cleanup of contaminated waste sites. It also confers liability on all involved with the waste site, even if they did not directly cause the contamination. Under CERCLA, hospitals have had to help pay for cleanup of waste sites to which they have sent their wastes.
- *The Superfund Amendments and Reauthorization Act (SARA) of 1986.* This act reauthorizes and strengthens CERCLA. In addition, Title III of SARA establishes a system of response in the event of an environmental disaster. Title III gives some hospitals additional environmental responsibilities (see chapter 6).
- *Infectious Waste Guidelines.* In 1986, the EPA published guidelines for the handling, treatment, and disposal of infectious waste. These are merely guidelines and do not possess the force of law. Because of well-publicized medical waste dumpings and societal concerns, however, the EPA has announced that it will reconsider its policy of just publishing guidelines on this subject.

Taken together, these EPA laws and guidelines represent a broad base of responsibility for health care facilities (see table 2-2, on p. 23). As is evident from the rules that have been strengthened, reauthorized, or reconsidered, EPA regulations are expanding and changing almost daily.

Although the EPA is a major source of regulatory control, it can also act as an excellent source of guidance and information. The Environmental Protection Agency publishes informative guides to help facilities understand and comply with regulations, such as its 1986 publication entitled *Understanding the Small Quantity Generator Hazardous Waste Rules: A Handbook for Small Businesses* and its *EPA Guide for Infectious Waste Management.* The regional or national offices of the EPA can be contacted to obtain copies of their material or for further information. Table 2-3 (see p. 24) lists the EPA regional offices.

U.S. Environmental Protection Agency, Office of Solid Waste and Emergency Response, Washington, DC 20460, 202/382-4700.

Centers for Disease Control

The Centers for Disease Control (CDC) safeguards the health of the American people by controlling and preventing disease. It conducts research and publishes results—most often in the *Morbidity and Mortality Weekly Report.* This periodical is an up-to-date and thorough reference for health care facilities that want to stay ahead of new guidelines and regulations on such topics as infection control, infectious waste, and worker protection from blood-borne infectious diseases such as AIDS and hepatitis B virus. Various agencies, such as the Joint Commission, OSHA, and the EPA, rely on the research and guidelines of the CDC.

The Centers for Disease Control has six operational units:

- *The Center for Environmental Health* works to control environmentally related and chronic diseases.
- *The Center for Health Promotion and Education* responds to the growing need for disease prevention and promotion of good health.
- *The Center for Prevention Services* cooperates with state and local health agencies on preventive health services.
- *The National Institute for Occupational Safety and Health (NIOSH)* recommends occupational safety and health standards and provides research, training, and technical assistance to promote healthful working conditions. The Occupational Safety and Health Administration relies heavily on NIOSH research in writing new regulations. In addition, NIOSH can be an excellent resource for the employee accident prevention element of safety.
- *The Center for Professional Development and Training* coordinates training to build a national work force committed to disease prevention and control. (This is another resource for facilities.)
- *The Center for Infectious Diseases* coordinates a national program to investigate, prevent, and control infectious disease. The Centers for Disease Control's infection control guidelines originate here.

Through these six centers, the CDC provides a wide variety of technical information and support services. Health care facilities should avail themselves of the CDC's numerous resources.

Centers for Disease Control, 1600 Clifton Road, N.E., Atlanta, GA 30333, 404/329-3311.

U.S. Food and Drug Administration

The Food and Drug Administration (FDA) is charged with supervising the development, testing, and monitoring of food and drug products and medical equipment. The Food and Drug Administration requires health care facilities to take corrective action to protect the safety and well-being of patients, staff, and visitors whenever information on a hazardous product is brought to a facility's attention. It is the responsibility of the facility to obtain, evaluate, and act upon all information concerning hazards of the equipment, food, and medication it uses.

Until the mid-1970s, the FDA had no well-defined control over medical devices. In 1976, the Medical Device Amendments to the Federal Food, Drug and

Cosmetics Act (which established the FDA) set up an FDA Bureau of Medical Devices (BMD). The Bureau of Medical Devices possesses the authority to ban or recall products that present a substantial and unreasonable risk for causing harm. The severity of the hazard determines whether the product is removed from the marketplace. If the risk is not severe enough to recall the product, the manufacturer still must notify users of the hazard(s).

Depending on the situation, products are recalled through letters, postcards, and telegrams. The Food and Drug Administration may require the manufacturer to send a "return-receipt" letter to the facility. This is a document that, when signed by an authorized employee of the facility, officially acknowledges that the facility has received the recall notice. It then becomes the facility's responsibility to initiate an organized procedure to communicate the necessary information to all appropriate staff and make arrangements to replace the product, if necessary. If the facility does not take some measures and the recalled product causes a serious accident, much of the liability may be transferred to the facility.

The Food and Drug Administration has also established the Medical Device and Laboratory Product Problem Reporting Program, whereby health care workers can report problems they find in the products they use. This program is geared toward improving communication of hazards resulting from medical products. For further information, contact Practicioner Reporting System, United States Pharmacopoeia, 12601 Twinbrook Parkway, Rockville, MD 20852, 800/638-6725.

Other sources of information on food, drug, or medical device hazards include the *FDA Enforcement Report,* available from the Press Office, Food and Drug Administration, 5600 Fishers Lane, Rockville, MD 20857; and the *Health Device Alerts,* available from Emergency Care Research Institute, 5200 Butler Pike, Plymouth Meeting, PA 19462.

U.S. Food and Drug Administration, 5600 Fishers Lane, Rockville, MD 20857, 301/443-1544.

U.S. Nuclear Regulatory Commission

The Nuclear Regulatory Commission (NRC) oversees the operation of nuclear power facilities and regulates the handling, use, and disposal of radioactive materials. Hospitals may use radiological substances in several areas of operation: nuclear medicine, radiology, clinical laboratories, and research laboratories. The types of materials used in hospitals usually result in low-level radioactive waste.

Radioactive waste is unlike infectious and hazardous waste in that the danger of the waste can only be completely removed by time. Over time, radioactive materials decay and become less hazardous. The rate of radioactive decay, called the half-life, can be very slow; some materials require thousands of years to become thoroughly harmless. Meanwhile, these substances emit dangerous radiation, which has been associated with cancers, birth defects, and other health problems.

As a result, these materials must be carefully handled during use and adequately contained for disposal. Hazardousness and half-lives vary widely among radiological materials, as do disposal techniques. Contaminated materials may be incinerated, put in a landfill, allowed to decay in storage, or disposed of through the sanitary sewer, depending on their type and the applicable regulations. The Nuclear Regulatory Commission has published regulations governing these practices in its *Standards for Protection Against Radiation.*

U.S. Nuclear Regulatory Commission, 1717 H Street, Washington, DC 20555, 301/492-7000.

State Requirements

Individual states have requirements for health care facilities on many of the same topics as federal agency regulations. However, the state requirements may be more rigorous or extensive than federal standards. These state rules are usually enforced through licensure or the periodic inspection and relicensure process. States may legislate practices in many areas, including the following:

- *Occupational safety and health.* Federal OSHA gives states the option of implementing their own workplace safety and health programs rather than adopting the federal program. State OSHA programs must be at least as stringent as the federal program.
- *Hazardous waste.* States may establish their own EPA hazardous waste management agencies to assist in compliance with EPA rules and possibly expand on them.
- *Infectious waste.* Although this is rapidly changing, the greatest source of rule making for infectious waste is state agencies. Regulations are usually issued by the board of health or state EPA, if there is one. In addition, local sewer districts may have rules for the disposal of hazardous or infectious materials through the sewer.
- *Workers' compensation.* A common denominator for all states is the existence of workers' compensation laws, which are generally enforced by the state's attorney general or an agency that handles similar matters. The penalties for failure to comply with these laws, as well as the actual compensation to injured employees, are cumulative and can cause financial hardship for any size facility. Effective accident prevention and comprehensive safety programs can minimize unreasonable workers' compensation costs.
- *Fire and health codes.* The state or local fire authority, normally the fire marshal's office, verifies that fire safety requirements are met using its own state codes and National Fire Protection Association (NFPA) codes. In addition, health or fire department officials, or the authority having jurisdiction, will verify compliance with required infection control techniques, sanitation practices, proper storage and disposal of hazardous materials, and training of staff in proper identification and control of hazardous substances.

Because state and local requirements on these and other subjects may differ from or expand upon national standards, it is crucial that health care facilities know the regulations that may affect them. As with federal mandates, facilities should be aware that regional requirements may change as new information becomes available. Abiding by state and local rules can provide a strong foundation for compliance with federal and voluntary standards.

□ Voluntary Compliance Agencies

Just as there have always been nonprofit health care facilities that have, in a way, "volunteered" medical services to the community, a parallel trend has also existed in health care—voluntary agencies have set standards for the health care industry. These agencies and their standards are highly regarded, and their accreditation of a facility is often evidence that the facility places high priority on safety and health.

Voluntary agencies act out of a sincere desire to enhance patient care and to ensure that the facility is a safe environment for its inhabitants. Moreover, many governmental agencies look to these voluntary groups for technical assistance in developing regulations for the health care industry. When incorporated into federal, state, or local regulations, voluntary standards become compulsory.

The Joint Commission, the National Fire Protection Association, the American National Standards Institute, and the Compressed Gas Association represent just a few of the many helpful voluntary organizations, which are too numerous to mention. Trade groups exist for practically every health care facility safety topic imaginable, and many states or regions have their own health care associations. Health care facilities are urged to make use of the many professional resources available to them. A brief list of suggested organizations appears in appendix A.

Joint Commission on Accreditation of Healthcare Organizations

With the growth of the voluntary compliance movement, regional and national health care associations appeared across the country. In 1951 several of these groups, including the American Hospital Association and the American Medical Association, founded the Joint Commission on Accreditation of Healthcare Organizations (Joint Commission). The purpose of the Joint Commission is to standardize practices and ensure at least a minimum standard for the quality of care for patients in American health care facilities.

Toward these ends, the Joint Commission developed an accreditation process based on surveys and compliance with standards. These standards, along with general suggestions for rendering high-quality patient care, appear in the Joint Commission's *Accreditation Manual for Hospitals,* which is published annually. This manual has many helpful suggestions for what should be included in an overall safety program, including accident prevention techniques, safety committee requirements, and fire safety recommendations. In developing many of its inspection criteria, the Joint Commission incorporates the standards of other agencies, such as the EPA, OSHA, and NFPA. Compliance with these federal rules provides the foundation for Joint Commission accreditation.

Any health care facility can apply to the Joint Commission for accreditation once certain preliminary requirements have been met. After the facility has paid the appropriate fees and completed the extensive preparatory materials, a Joint Commission team will conduct a survey for accreditation. If most standards are met and the facility is substantially in compliance, it will receive accreditation for three years.

The entire process of Joint Commission accreditation can be beneficial, although it is somewhat time-consuming and relatively expensive. The value it holds will have to be assessed by each facility. Should the facility decide to proceed, it will have behind it the full consulting resources of this respected, non-profit group that is recognized as a source of excellence by many federal, state, and local governments and their safety-related departments. In addition, through the accreditation process, health care personnel will learn effective means of limiting risks, lowering financial losses, and improving patient care.

If seeking accreditation is not feasible, another approach is to use the Joint Commission's accreditation manual's guidelines in the facility and to make them part of the comprehensive safety program. By using the manual, the facility can rely on the technical knowledge and expertise of the Joint Commission in meeting safety requirements.

Joint Commission on Accreditation of Healthcare Organizations, 875 N. Michigan Avenue, Chicago, IL 60611, 312/642-6061.

National Fire Protection Association

The National Fire Protection Association (NFPA) is an independent, nonprofit organization that codifies fire safety standards for the construction of all buildings in the country, including health care facilities. The organization draws on expert advice from various fields in developing its codes, and it is widely recognized as a reliable source of fire protection guidance. Consequently, codes have been accepted by the federal government and most state and local governments as the basis for their fire prevention and construction codes. The Joint Commission also exchanges information with NFPA through active participation on NFPA committees.

The two most important standards for health care facilities are NFPA 99, *Standard for Health Care Facilities,* and NFPA 101, *Life Safety Code.* NFPA 99 establishes criteria for safeguarding patients and health care personnel from fire, explosion, and electrical and related hazards associated with locations where anesthesia is administered. (NFPA 99 is part of more than 50 publications that apply to health care facilities.) The sections of NFPA 99 that more specifically apply to health care facilities are Respiratory Therapy, Essential Electrical Systems for Health Care Facilities, Safe Use of Electricity in Patient Areas of Hospitals, Health Care Emergency Preparedness, Laboratories in Health Related Institutions, Medical-Surgical Vacuum Systems in Hospitals, and Use of Inhalation Anesthetics (Flammable & Nonflammable).

NFPA 101 establishes the codes for life safety by considering a number of elements such as early warning detection and alarm systems, fire partitions, exit identification and lighting, sprinkler systems, building care maintenance, and storage for all occupied buildings. Included in the code are requirements for emergency preparedness plans and drills, exit arrangements, portable fire extinguishers, and waste handling systems. The disaster preparedness section provides information necessary for the preparation and implementation of a facility's individual plan.

(*Note:* In some areas of the South and Midwest the Uniform Fire Code (UFC) sometimes supersedes NFPA codes. Those for whom this might apply should check with their local and state regulatory agencies.)

One of the best sources of overall information on the latest developments in fire protection systems, equipment, and techniques is the latest edition of the NFPA *Fire Protection Handbook.* Also, an NFPA training film, *Fire Safety in Health Care Facilities,* provides an overview of fire protection methods for health care. Another NFPA film, *Evacuation of Medical Facilities,* focuses on successful evacuations from a health care facility.

The National Fire Protection Association is also an excellent source of training materials including books, pamphlets, posters, slide programs, films, and training manuals for both in-house and home fire protection training. In addition, a number of seminars are offered each year, and technical advice is available. An individual membership is beneficial for the person most responsible for the fire-safety function in each facility.

National Fire Protection Association, Batterymarch Park, Quincy, MA 02269, 800/344-3555.

American National Standards Institute

In 1918, several professional organizations and government agencies formed the American National Standards Institute (ANSI) to coordinate the issuance of standards by agencies with similar responsibilities. The goal of ANSI is to minimize duplication and conflict between the numerous regulations affecting business and industry. The organization works to assist voluntary and governmental agencies in developing regulations while seeking a consensus on the need for standards.

The American National Standards Institute conducts a review process by which a regulation or requirement is approved as an American National Standard. In order to achieve this approval, the agency issuing the standard must be able to provide evidence that all those affected by the standard were allowed either to participate in or comment on the development of the regulation. With this approval, the standard is then generally recognized and accepted for use.

American National Standards Institute approval extends to regulations affecting health care as well. Through its approval process, ANSI ensures that when the health care industry is affected by a regulation it has a say in the standard's development. Health care managers and administrators should make use of this opportunity to contribute to the process by which standards that directly affect them are developed.

American National Standards Institute, 1430 Broadway, New York, NY 10018, 212/354-3300.

Compressed Gas Association

Health care facilities routinely use a number of compressed gases, including ethylene oxide, anesthetic gases, and oxygen. As these gases are stored under tremendous pressure, even minimal disturbance can cause this pressure to be released in a destructive manner. If not handled and stored with great caution, compressed gases pose a serious danger of explosion, injury, and property damage.

The Compressed Gas Association (CGA) was founded in 1913 as a nonprofit trade association representing the compressed gas industries. It provides technical advice and safety coordination for businesses in these industries. However, the CGA is also concerned with the handling of compressed gases wherever they are used, including health care facilities. The Compressed Gas Association provides a variety of services to users of compressed gases, including technical publications and audiovisual materials, and it advises NFPA in developing compressed gas standards. The Compressed Gas Association is an excellent source of information on the safe use of compressed gases.

Compressed Gas Association, Inc., 1235 Jefferson Davis Highway, Arlington, VA 22202, 703/979-0900.

☐ Comparing Applicable Regulations

As has been stated, the voluntary standards and governmental regulations affecting health care are many and various. (Table 2-4 on p. 25 summarizes the agencies discussed in this chapter and the scope of their services.) Requirements are often duplicated by several agencies, and sometimes different agencies may publish rules or guidelines that are in conflict with each other. Compounding the problem is the rapid pace at which some requirements grow and change, particularly in the hazardous/infectious waste area.

The sheer number and complexity of requirements become less threatening, however, if viewed from the right perspective. Many of the regulations overlap because the responsibilities of the various agencies overlap. For example, both the CDC and the EPA publish guidelines on infectious waste management, and NFPA codes are integrated into Joint Commission accreditation criteria. Discrepancies may be caused by new problems requiring new regulations, such as those for hazardous and infectious materials (for example, states rushing to catch up with ever-changing federal hazardous waste regulations). Governmental agencies are learning to work together in an attempt to avoid or correct such conflicting standards.

☐ Conclusion

Most compliance organizations work to make information and assistance available to those who need it. Many regulatory officials realize that their standards may seem confusing and try to enhance understanding through publications, training, and direct mailings. These agencies can also be contacted by mail or telephone with questions or concerns, and many agencies operate hotlines on specific topics. Concerned personnel who take the time to use the many resources available will find these regulations less intimidating and compliance an achievable goal.

Table 2-1. OSHA Regional Offices

Region	Geographical Area Covered	OSHA Regional Office
I	Connecticut,* Maine, Massachusetts, New Hampshire, Rhode Island, Vermont*	16–18 North Street 1 Dock Square Building 4th Floor Boston, MA 02109 Telephone: 617/565-1161
II	New Jersey, New York,* Puerto Rico	201 Varick Street 6th Floor New York, NY 10014 Telephone: 212/337-2325
III	Delaware, District of Columbia, Maryland,* Pennsylvania, Virginia,* West Virginia	Gateway Building, Suite 2100 3535 Market Street Philadelphia, PA 19104 Telephone: 212/596-1201
IV	Alabama, Florida, Georgia, Kentucky,* Mississippi, North Carolina,* South Carolina,* Tennessee*	1375 Peachtree Street, N.E. Suite 587 Atlanta, GA 30367 Telephone: 404/347-3573
V	Illinois, Indiana,* Michigan,* Minnesota,* Ohio, Wisconsin	230 South Dearborn Street 32nd Floor, Room 3244 Chicago, IL 60604 Telephone: 312/353-2200
VI	Arkansas, Louisiana, New Mexico,* Oklahoma, Texas	525 Griffin Street Room 602 Dallas, TX 75202 Telephone: 214/767-3731
VII	Iowa,* Kansas, Missouri, Nebraska	911 Walnut Street, Room 406 Kansas City, MO 64106 Telephone: 816/374-5861
VIII	Colorado, Montana, North Dakota, South Dakota, Utah,* Wyoming*	Federal Building, Room 1576 1961 Stout Street Denver, CO 80294 Telephone: 303/844-3061
IX	Arizona,* California,* Hawaii,* Nevada*	71 Stevenson Street 4th Floor San Francisco, CA 94105 Telephone: 415/995-5672
X	Alaska,* Idaho,* Oregon,* Washington*	Federal Office Building Room 6003 909 First Avenue Seattle, WA 98174 Telephone: 206/442-5930

*These states and territories operate their own OSHA-approved job safety and health programs (except Connecticut and New York, whose plans cover public employees only).

Table 2-2. Laws Empowering the EPA

Law	Allows EPA to:
1. Clean Air Act, 1970	Set permissible levels for hazardous and visible emissions into the air.
2. Clean Water Act, 1977 (reauthorized 1987)	Limit discharge of pollutants into waterways. Set up the NPDES.*
3. Toxic Substances Control Act, 1976	Regulate manufacture, distribution, and use of toxic chemicals.
4. Resource Conservation and Recovery Act, 1976	Establish system by which wastes are tracked from "cradle to grave."
5. Comprehensive Environmental Response, Compensation, and Liability Act, 1980 (also known as Superfund)	Set aside funds for cleanup of contaminated waste sites. Broaden liability for contaminated sites.
6. Superfund Amendments and Reauthorization Act, 1986	Reauthorize CERCLA. Establish system of response for environmental disasters.

*NPDES = National Pollutant Discharge Elimination System.

Table 2-3. EPA Regional Offices

Region	Geographical Area Covered	U.S. EPA Regional Office
I	Connecticut, Maine, Massachusetts, New Hampshire, Rhode Island, Vermont	State Waste Programs Branch JFK Federal Building Boston, MA 02203
II	New Jersey, New York, Puerto Rico, Virgin Islands	Air and Waste Management Division 26 Federal Plaza New York, NY 10278
III	Delaware, District of Columbia, Maryland, Pennsylvania, Virginia, West Virginia	Waste Management Branch MS 3HW 34 841 Chestnut Street Philadelphia, PA 19107
IV	Alabama, Florida, Georgia, Kentucky, Mississippi, North Carolina, South Carolina, Tennessee	Hazardous Waste Management Division 345 Courtland Street, N.E. Atlanta, GA 30365
V	Illinois, Indiana, Michigan, Minnesota, Ohio, Wisconsin	RCRA Activities Waste Management Division P.O. Box A3587 Chicago, IL 60690
VI	Arkansas, Louisiana, New Mexico, Oklahoma, Texas	Air and Hazardous Materials Division 1201 Elm Street Inter-First Two Building Dallas, TX 75270
VII	Iowa, Kansas, Nebraska, Missouri	RCRA Branch 726 Minnesota Avenue Kansas City, KS 66620
VIII	Colorado, Montana, North Dakota, South Dakota, Utah, Wyoming	Waste Management Division (8 HWM-ON) One Denver Place, Suite 1300 999 18th Street Denver, CO 80202-2413
IX	Arizona, California, Hawaii, Nevada, American Samoa, Guam	Toxics and Waste Management Division 215 Fremont Street San Francisco, CA 94105
X	Alaska, Idaho, Oregon, Washington	Waste Management Branch—MS-530 1200 Sixth Avenue Seattle, WA 98101

Table 2-4. Summary of Agencies and Their Scope

Governmental Agency	Scope
1. Occupational Safety and Health Administration (OSHA)	Workplace safety and health
2. U.S. Environmental Protection Agency (EPA)	Control of the release of harmful materials into the environment
3. Centers for Disease Control (CDC)	Control and prevention of disease
4. U.S. Food and Drug Administration (FDA)	Supervision of the development, testing, and monitoring of food, drugs, and medical devices
5. U.S. Nuclear Regulatory Commission (NRC)	The handling, use and disposal of radiological materials
6. State and local agencies	Workers' compensation; many areas also covered by federal agencies
Voluntary Agency	**Scope**
1. Joint Commission on Accreditation of Healthcare Organizations (Joint Commission)	Standardization of practices to ensure high-quality patient care; accreditation
2. National Fire Protection Association (NFPA)	Prevention of fire through standards and technical support
3. American National Standards Institute (ANSI)	Coordination and approval of standards
4. Compressed Gas Association (CGA)	Services to users of compressed gases

Chapter 3
Building an Effective Safety Committee

Safety committees are suggested or required by at least two compliance agencies. Specifically, the Occupational Safety and Health Administration (OSHA) recommends them to review accidents, develop safety motivational programs, and assist in policy development. Other groups, such as state and local agencies, together with OSHA, view the existence of an effective safety committee as evidence of the employer's desire to ensure that employees have a safe and healthful working environment. Safety committees are also required in Joint Commission on Accreditation of Healthcare Organizations (Joint Commission) standards, which specify certain elements that must be included and personnel who should participate.

The safety committee is more than just a regulatory precaution. It can and should be a group that makes the difference between a safe environment and a hazardous one, between money saved and money needlessly spent. The safety committee has this potential because it assists in developing, implementing, and evaluating many crucial safety functions. It serves as the centralized advisory group to the safety director, chief executive officer (CEO), and administrators, who will often act on the results of safety committee reviews and on the group's suggestions.

At the same time, the safety committee can spark an active interest in safety among employees. Including both employee and management representation helps employees feel that they have an important role to play in safety; these committee members will then convey their enthusiasm to their coworkers. As other employees have a chance to sit on the committee, commitment and a willingness to participate actively in safety concerns will spread among employees. It is the workers' support and involvement that contribute most to the success of safety programs.

The safety committee serves as a clearinghouse for important safety-related documents that might otherwise be filed away and not be reviewed or acted upon. This is particularly true for incident reports because the safety committee evaluates statistics based on recent reports. Most significantly, the group solicits advice from employees and suggests corrective actions so that the problems that cause incidents are not left to grow into major hazards. In addition, the committee evaluates and revises policies and procedures to reflect changing needs and requirements. Keeping the policies and procedures current is important so that they can continue to fulfill their role as the written foundation for the safety program.

Finally, the safety committee is involved in training and motivation. Suggesting ideas for training, planning in-services, and perhaps even conducting the training are additional responsibilities for safety committee members. As they discover hazards both through their experience on the committee and through their everyday work, committee members will be able to suggest areas to target in training. Creative members can also plan ways to increase the effectiveness of departmental in-service education and incentive programs. The CEO and the safety director should treat the committee as a valuable creative resource, consisting of people who possess hands-on experience with what works and what does not work.

□ The Safety Director

As explained in chapter 1, both the safety committee and the overall safety program must have direction and coordination. In the past, the responsibility for directing the safety program was often delegated to the engineering or housekeeping department. Although health care engineers are knowledgeable about the facility and can undergo further safety training, the direction of the safety program should really be viewed as a professional task in and of itself, requiring specific education and experience. The Joint Commission specifically requires the CEO to appoint a safety director who is qualified for the position by training or experience. As risks escalate and safety becomes more technical, the qualifications for the position of safety director will become more sophisticated.

Depending on the needs and size of the facility, the job of directing the safety program may require varying amounts of staff time. Some smaller facilities may decide to appoint an employee who also holds another position. A larger facility's needs may require that one or more full-time employees act in this capacity. Regardless of the staff time devoted to directing the program, it is important to remember not to overtax the safety director if that person also has other responsibilities within the facility.

Much of the concern regarding the appointment of a safety director relates to the expense involved as measured against what are perceived to be limited benefits. However, like the safety program in general, having a safety director must be viewed as a long-term investment. Benefits may not be evident immediately. By the very nature of the safety director's job (*preventing* losses), it may be difficult to measure the direct effects. An accident that was prevented, for example, will never appear on a report or statistic. This is not to say, however, that the safety director's impact will not be demonstrable. A qualified and experienced director should possess the skills not only to reduce risks but to provide evidence of his or her work as well.

The specific responsibilities involved in the safety director's position, like any other job, may differ depending on the health care facility. Basically, they consist of tasks involved in providing leadership to the safety program, such as working with the safety committee on accident trends and inspections, keeping policies and procedures current and effective, maintaining a liaison with departments, serving on multiple facility committees, coordinating fire and disaster drills, and helping design motivational programs for safety. As part of this leadership role, the safety director also advises and consults with the administration on safety matters.

The CEO must ensure that the safety director has the authority necessary to carry out all of his or her responsibilities. The naming of the safety director should be publicized as an important appointment, demonstrating top management's faith in the person chosen. The CEO should explicitly state, perhaps in a facilitywide communication, that the director has been granted the authority necessary to carry out the job.

☐ Committee Leadership and Authority

The safety director should work closely with the safety committee. In fact, in some facilities the director also serves as chairperson of the committee. However, such an arrangement may not always be advisable. Not only will it add another obligation to an already crowded schedule, but it may also centralize decision making to the extent that the full range of ideas and alternatives is not always considered. A committee chairperson who is not involved so extensively in steering the safety program can offer a fresh, perhaps less biased, perspective. This approach also gives the other experienced committee members the opportunity to be chairperson. The rotation of chairpersons and the diversity of ideas and attitudes it brings enhance the quality of group decisions.

According to Joint Commission standards, upon formation of the safety committee, the committee's authority must be approved in writing by the governing body or CEO (or someone the CEO designates) and the medical staff. The approval is necessary so that action can be taken when conditions exist that pose an immediate threat to life or risk of damage to the equipment or building.

After approval has been granted, the CEO or designee appoints the chairperson. The chairperson should be knowledgeable in his or her field as well as in safety and, preferably, should have experience serving on a safety committee. The chairperson has the following duties:

- Devise a schedule for meetings.
- Arrange for a place to convene.
- Notify members of meetings.
- Plan the agenda.
- Review the minutes and materials for the meeting.
- Obtain any speakers or instructors for the meeting.
- Lead and facilitate the discussion during the meeting.
- Ensure that safety committee activities and successes are publicized within the facility.

Many facilities rotate chairpersons every year or two to increase participation and avoid burnout. Although terms should last long enough to allow the chairperson to build experience, rotation will afford a greater number of people the opportunity to learn through leadership.

In order to expedite committee activities and maintain necessary documentation, the committee should also have a secretary. The secretary should be experienced and dependable, with a demonstrated desire to participate in safety matters. The secretary will be responsible for these tasks:

- Prepare and distribute the agenda and the minutes.
- Document the status of committee recommendations.
- Report this information to the committee.
- Assist the chairperson in any work, as requested.

The safety director and committee chairperson should both work to grant this appointment some measure of prestige.

☐ Committee Composition

Other than the secretary and the chairperson, the safety committee must have representation from several departments and levels in the facility hierarchy. The Joint Commission requires the CEO or designee to appoint the committee members. An effective safety committee might include the following members:

- Administration representative
- Medical staff representative
- Nursing representative(s)
- Director of maintenance (or engineering, or both)
- Supervisory representatives (one or two on rotation)
- Director of housekeeping
- Director of dietary
- Human resources representative
- Directors of safety and security
- Labor representative (if there is a union)
- Risk management representative
- Three nonsupervisory employees (rotated periodically)

The goal of this specific composition is to ensure a *multidisciplinary* committee. Revisions in the past few years in Joint Commission requirements have made the standards less prescriptive; that is, they no longer specify the exact composition of the committee. Instead, commission accreditation surveyors look for a committee with wide-ranging representation, with emphasis on representatives from the administration and clinical and support services. The members previously required by the Joint Commission may figure prominently in this broad base, but others should also be chosen to build a multidisciplinary committee. Figure 3-1 (see p. 36) graphically represents the multidisciplinary approach.

Larger facilities may expand on this minimum membership and include representatives from such departments as infection control, quality assurance, employee health, and pathology. For all facilities, the structure of the safety committee should embrace individuals from all areas of operation who are willing to participate. Members must possess the enthusiasm and commitment to develop, implement, and maintain a comprehensive, facilitywide safety program.

The committee's size should probably be limited to approximately 15 members. Many more than that will cause the group to become unwieldy and unproductive. Very large organizations may want to maintain two safety committees, each with its own clearly defined set of responsibilities, in order to avoid the pitfalls of one excessively large, unmanageable body.

In addition, like the chairperson of the committee, some members should be rotated, particularly supervisors and employees. They should have a defined term of service of which they are advised in advance. Rotation attracts members with new ideas and fresh motivation. It also gives a greater number of staff members the opportunity to participate in high-level safety functions, thus extending the commitment to safety to more of those primarily responsible for carrying out the program. All of the rotations, however, should not occur simultaneously. Terms of membership should be staggered to keep experienced members on the committee at all times.

☐ Members' Responsibilities

In any group setting, it is essential to clarify the role of each participant. Members of the safety committee should have a set of guidelines and responsibilities that they can refer to as they begin their involvement with the committee. They must know that work will be required of them because their input and assistance is valuable to the organization.

Because the committee is a multidisciplinary unit, its membership may represent a spectrum of personal and professional backgrounds. Members may range from department heads to administrators to employees. Some may represent labor, others management. Some members will bring concerns specific to their departments, others more generalized objectives. Regardless of the individual's unique situation, all members should be directed to forgo personal motives as much as possible in favor of the goals of the committee as a whole. Although individual and departmental problems will be considered, the safety standard must always reflect facility, employee, and patient safety.

Beyond this duty to remain objective, the members must also protect the confidentiality of what is said in safety committee meetings. The chairperson should assure all members that what is expressed during meetings will be kept strictly confidential. Only through this type of assurance will members feel free to speak candidly. This rule of confidentiality should be strictly enforced.

Another member responsibility includes participating actively in safety committee business. Members should contribute insight gained from experience and training. Of course, members must attend all meetings.

Member responsibilities also include the following:

- Report any unsafe conditions that they detect or that others have reported to them.
- Review summaries of recent incident reports.
- Participate in investigations and inspections.
- Contribute ideas and suggestions for improvement.
- Act as models of sound safety practices for other employees.
- Provide written reports on unsafe procedures and individual actions contrary to safe conduct.
- Report exemplary employee behavior.
- Help sponsor contests, safety drives, incentive programs, and so forth.

Figure 3-2 (see p. 37) summarizes the basic responsibilities of safety committee participants. Members should be chosen based on their ability to fulfill these duties. When beginning a term of service, the members should be invited to meet with the chairperson, who will explain their roles and provide a written list of specific responsibilities. This meeting is also an excellent opportunity for the chairperson to welcome new members and answer any questions.

☐ Goals and Objectives

The basic goal of the safety committee—the foundation on which all its activities rest—is to help provide a safe environment for the facility and staff, thereby contributing to a high-quality patient care environment. This goal is necessarily broad. It outlines the safety advisory function of the committee and presents this function as a step toward the facility's primary aim: impeccable patient care. Presenting the committee's activities in this light helps members see the far-reaching influence of their work.

This generalized goal translates to four specific objectives that every safety committee should adopt. These objectives should be recognized and documented so that members can keep sight of the role of the committee:

1. *Provide technical support to the safety director and administrator.* Through its collective training and experience, the committee is an excellent advisory group, offering the director and administrator technical information and practical tips.
2. *Adequately respond to recognized safety problems.* This is accomplished through the review of many documents, including:

   - Incident reports
   - Inspection results
   - Safety policies and procedures
   - Accident investigation results

   In addition to reviewing these records, as part of their troubleshooting role committee members also solicit opinions, concerns, and suggestions from the employees in their departments. Their recommendations will help the committee achieve its objective of adequately reviewing and responding to safety problems.
3. *Promote a facilitywide concern for safety.* Many safety committees can become so mired in paperwork and technical review that they lose sight of the overwhelming human element in safety. Safety programs are carried out by individuals, people with needs and concerns. A major objective for the safety committee should focus on involving and motivating the hospital's staff. This goal can be accomplished in a variety of ways—through training, in-house publications, incentive programs, and other safety campaigns. Only through actively pursuing employee commitment can the safety committee successfully fulfill its principal goal of helping ensure comprehensive safety in the facility.
4. *Serve as a safety resource and advisory group.* Finally, the safety committee must strive to be accessible to employees and managers as a resource for safety information and assistance. When employees voice a safety concern or would like to discuss ideas for improvement, the committee should take the time to hear their views. Members should listen with interest and consider the suggestions presented. In this way, an equivalent responsibility to employees complements the committee's obligation to the administration. By providing a forum for employees' ideas, committee participants generate the feeling among employees that the committee and, by extension, the administration, cares about their anxiety, knowledge, and suggestions.

☐ Safety Committee Functions

When all the technicalities of composition and responsibility are determined, the safety committee can begin to tackle the tasks required to meet its objectives. The committee is expected to handle the following tasks:

- *Review the policies and procedures that establish safety standards for the facility.* Keeping these documents current is crucial to maintaining a safety program that can adapt to the changing needs of the facility.

- *Develop in-service training on safety for employees.* Training will not only upgrade the safety competence of the staff but will also help employees realize that safety goals are attainable.
- *Establish procedures for acting on employee suggestions.* The committee should implement a standardized process for immediately responding to employee ideas and concerns. The committee should thank the employee, explain the status of the problem, and outline the action that can be taken. Committee members must follow up on any assurances they make to employees.
- *Consider new federal, state, and local requirements so that procedures and facility regulations continue to comply.* Guidelines and regulations change frequently to improve safety and health program management. Complying with these requirements will also help the facility save money by preventing avoidable losses.
- *Review and evaluate accident reports (or summaries of recent incidents).* The review must be documented, along with the action taken or recommended.
- *Conduct systematic inspection tours to discover unsafe conditions and practices.* This includes surprise inspections that may yield a more realistic portrait of the everyday practices in the facility.
- *Promote the adoption and use of departmental safety regulations.* Both through their work on the committee and during performance of their individual jobs, safety committee members should function as supporters of safety procedures and models of proper risk avoidance.
- *Provide specific safety information to supervisors.* Supervisors can become a significant channel that the safety committee can use to disseminate information and support to employees.
- *Maintain a link with the administration in order to fulfill the safety committee's role as an advisory body.* The safety committee can function as a valuable managerial tool, and it should provide input to the administrative decision-making process.
- *Establish a hazard surveillance program within the facility and on its grounds.* For assistance in this function, the committee can rely on an often-overlooked resource: security personnel. Through proper training and cooperation, security officers can begin to detect safety lapses as well as security risks on their rounds. Maintenance personnel can also assist through preventive maintenance. In fact, in a supportive atmosphere, virtually all employees can become more alert to any unsafe conditions surrounding them.
- *Recommend improvements in personal protective clothing and equipment.* This is particularly important with the growing routine use of garments such as gloves and aprons to protect against infection by AIDS, hepatitis B, or other blood-borne infectious diseases. Personal protective equipment includes that used in support functions, such as goggles for operating dangerous machinery.
- *Implement a process to evaluate the safety program's progress.* The program should be regularly reviewed, reconsidered, and modernized.
- *Conduct regularly scheduled meetings.* Naturally, accomplishing these goals requires regular, well-planned meetings.

After gathering information gained as a result of these tasks, the safety committee will make specific recommendations. The Joint Commission requires that safety committee suggestions and actions be reported at least quarterly to the administrative, medical, and nursing staffs and others as appropriate. The facility must be able to provide evidence that these suggestions are evaluated by appropriate administrative directors of the areas affected and that follow-up action is documented in safety committee minutes.

The functions of the safety committee may seem to consist of an overwhelming number of duties. For that reason, the chairperson must set reasonable, attainable goals for the short term (three months, two months, or even for the intervals between meetings). People need to see the progress they are making, even though it may seem minimal in relation to the long-term goal.

Task Forces

Many committees have discovered that appointing task forces to deal with discrete, manageable assignments is an effective method for accomplishing several tasks simultaneously. This is particularly important when an overload of specific responsibilities begins to detract from the productivity of the safety committee. As an example, perhaps equipment failures in a number of areas are causing alarm. Task forces of two or three members (or even one member) from each affected area can be assigned to investigate specific failures. Then each task force documents its activities and reports back to the committee as a whole for further action. The point is that with some ingenuity, the dilemmas that are bound to occur in this group setting can be resolved.

Networking Committees

During goal setting and as they begin to initiate projects, safety committees often encounter an unexpected obstacle—tangled and confused relations with all of the other committees in the facility. In many health care facilities, this problem arises from an excess of committees—fire safety, risk management, disaster preparedness, quality assurance, infection control, utilization review.

Although some committees must remain separate to comply with regulations, others may be consolidated. Often, all quality assurance activities can be accomplished using one committee, as can all or most safety functions. In many facilities, the safety committee should be able to address accident prevention, hazardous waste, disaster preparedness, fire safety, and other safety issues without forming other committees.

In addition, to encourage coordination, the safety committee chairperson must maintain a liaison with the other committees, such as infection control, quality assurance, and radiation safety. The Joint Commission requires evidence of information exchange and consultation between the safety committee and any department safety programs as well as with the aforementioned committees.

□ Conducting Effective Committee Meetings

The most frequently asked question on the topic of safety committees is, How can I make my meetings more successful? Most people easily grasp the composition, goals, and functions of the committee but find the improvement of the actual meetings a perplexing problem. Frustration with committees is natural and, in fact, committees are notorious for their inefficiency and the corresponding lack of enthusiasm on the part of members.

A few tips and some common sense can at least set the committee off in the right direction. First, realize that lengthy and too-frequent meetings immediately turn people off. Meetings usually have the greatest success when held once a month (Joint Commission standards say at least every other month) for no longer than an hour. This avoids overloading members with either too many meetings or too few, which are interminable when finally held.

The meeting room should be large enough to accommodate everyone easily, and it must be comfortable, private, and free of distractions. Using the same site for every meeting will heighten members' comfort in familiar surroundings.

Because members must accomplish a great deal in their limited time, the chairperson and the secretary should be prepared. Thorough preparation for the planned business conserves time. One way to prepare is to develop a basic agenda that can be particularized for each meeting. The chairperson should send the agenda to members at least one week, preferably two weeks, in advance. The agenda alerts the members that a meeting is approaching. Members should be asked to contact the chairperson well in advance of the meeting if they want something placed on the agenda (figure 3-3 on p. 37 presents a sample agenda).

In addition, any supporting documentation, such as inspection results and the minutes of the previous meeting, should be distributed with the agenda so that members will have time to review information relevant to the next meeting. Sending out a calendar of meeting times, dates, and places at the beginning of the year can prevent overlapping, missed, or forgotten meetings. This may also enhance members' commitment to the long-term success of the committee.

Another way to add to the success of meetings is to vary the format occasionally by inviting knowledgeable and entertaining speakers. This way, the committee learns while also getting a break from its routine work. Another option for enlivening meetings is to offer refreshments. Some facilities have had great success with occasional appreciation lunches. The important fact to remember is that members should be rewarded for their efforts. A little pampering often goes a long way.

The committee chairperson can also do much to enhance the effectiveness of meetings. The chairperson should avoid, at all costs, an excessively demanding approach to members. They are volunteers devoting valuable time and effort to the program. In addition, the chairperson must facilitate, not monopolize, discussion. He or she should acknowledge contributions during the meetings and coax comments from those members who may be reluctant to speak out. Through adequate planning, a consistent format, and attention to motivating members, the committee chairperson can move appreciably toward a better functioning, more effective safety committee.

□ Labor–Management Cooperation

In unionized health care facilities, safety often becomes divided between management efforts and labor activities. This division often exacerbates dissension. A growing recognition of this problem has led to increasing labor–management cooperation on safety. In many cases, both parties hold similar goals for safety, such as fewer accidents or a more secure workplace. Safety committees can draw on these similarities by including both labor and management representatives, while also continuing to meet OSHA and Joint Commission requirements. United efforts can help the safety committee more completely identify vulnerabilities, reduce accidents and injuries, and improve productivity levels.

When establishing such a joint safety committee, the chairperson should stress to the members that both parties have much to gain from effective cooperation. However, members should also be advised that the committee is not an arena for debating differences but for discussing safety issues. To prevent disputes, the labor and management members should not be participating in contract negotiations while they are on the committee. This way, the committee is buffered from the collective bargaining process.

As with any committee participants, members must be chosen (by both labor and management) who are highly motivated toward making the workplace safer and more healthful. As the combined safety committee begins to perceive mutual objectives and assess the overall safety program, members will realize the value of being involved in such a bilateral effort. Members will take measurable steps toward understanding one another better while learning from each other along the way. In this way, joint labor–management safety committees can quell labor–management dissension while amplifying the success of the safety program.

☐ Conclusion

Although many facilities already have safety committees, these groups may not be achieving their full potential. Safety committees can serve as a valuable resource and advisory group, promoting and advancing safety. The key is to organize the committee and its functions, balance representation, and strive to motivate and reward its members. Reevaluating and perhaps restructuring the existing committee can provide numerous benefits. Whatever the status of the present committee, a renewed interest in conducting more successful meetings can boost performance. With some time and attention invested in this group, the safety committee can become an effective, adaptive force that sustains and guides a results-oriented safety program.

Figure 3-1. The Multidisciplinary Safety Committee

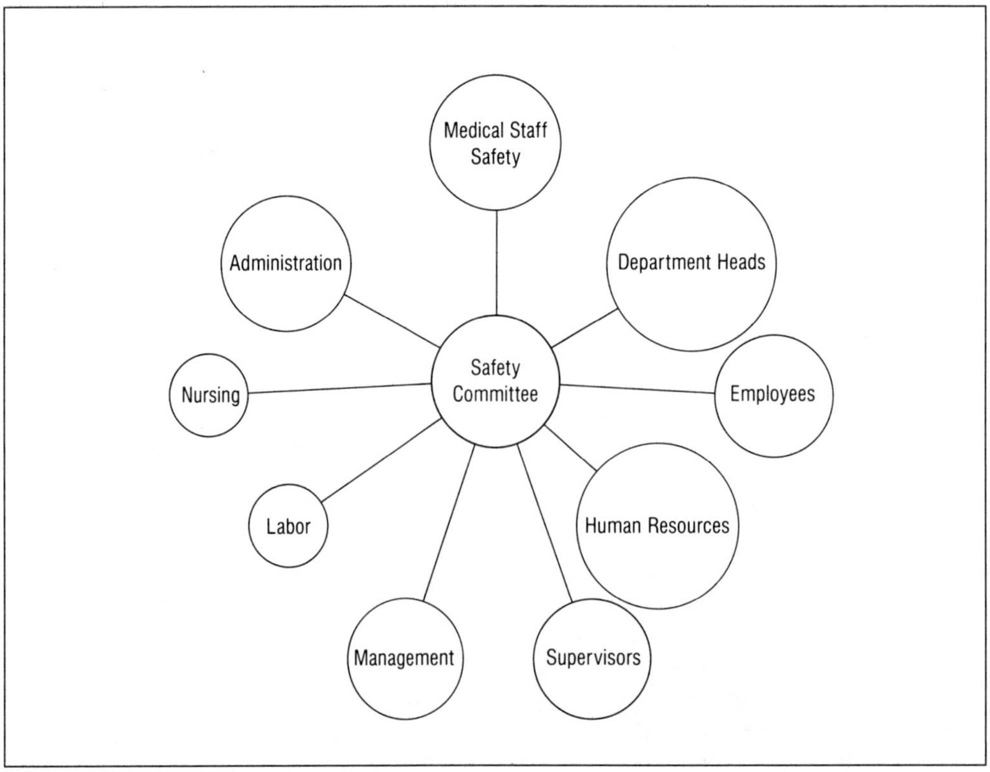

Figure 3-2. Responsibilities of Safety Committee Participants

Chairperson

- Schedule meetings.
- Arrange location.
- Notify members.
- Plan agenda.
- Prepare for meeting.
- Obtain any necessary speakers.
- Lead discussion.
- Publicize committee activities.

Secretary

- Prepare minutes and agenda.
- Distribute minutes.
- Document status of committee recommendations.
- Report these to committee.
- Assist the chairperson.

Member

- Remain objective.
- Guard confidentiality.
- Participate actively.
- Attend all meetings.
- Report safe and unsafe conditions.
- Contribute ideas and suggestions.
- Help in safety motivation.
- Assist in the ongoing evaluation of the safety program.

Figure 3-3. Sample Safety Committee Agenda

Date:
Time:
Place:
Roll call (list those present):
Reading of minutes from previous meeting:
Unfinished business from previous meeting:
Closure of any previous business (describe):
Discussion of new business. Topics could include:*

- Inspection reports
- Reports on safety training
- Incident trends and serious incidents
- Outstanding recommendations
- Evaluation of program effectiveness
- A speaker
- Revisions of safety policies and procedures
- Other safety concerns of the facility
- Incentive programs planned

Goal setting:
Date and time of next meeting:
Adjournment

---

*In order to allow adequate time to discuss each topic, only one or two subjects should be discussed at each meeting.

Chapter 4
Departmental Safety

Although the facilitywide safety program forms a coordinated, integrated whole, safety must begin at the departmental level. It is here that employees carry out the program's requirements and procedures. Safe actions and preventive measures at this level, outlined in specific departmental policies and procedures, have the greatest impact on the overall success of the safety program. Many departments have similar safety concerns that can be approached using basic safety concepts common to all such risks.

□ Hiring Safety-Conscious Employees

A program of employee safety begins during the hiring process. Along with the usual prerequisites such as adequate education and experience, a qualified candidate should also demonstrate concern for and knowledge of safety. Considering safety before an employee is hired will promote safe conditions even as the employee learns the job. Hiring safety-conscious employees provides a strong basis that the safety program can use to build on in training.

This trait of safety consciousness may be determined in various ways. The employee's previous safety record may serve as a clue. A record of unusually frequent accidents or excessive lost work time may represent cause for concern. It is also important to consider that a weak or nonexistent safety program at the employee's previous facility may have contributed to a poor safety record.

More information can be gained from talking with the employee about safety. Ask about the importance the applicant places on safety, and have applicants describe previous safety programs in which they have been involved. This discussion often can reveal the employee's potential commitment to safety.

Job descriptions should be developed that include safety requirements. These descriptions can then act as criteria for the selection of employees. Conduct a thorough interview, referring to the job description as a measurement of qualifications. During the interview, describe the job and its requirements in detail, targeting questions toward determining the applicant's intellectual and physical abilities to perform the job well and safely.

General hiring practices are important in acquiring safety-conscious employees. References, especially previous employers, should be checked. Licensing for many professions, such as pharmacy and anesthesiology, varies from state to state. Therefore, the applicant's license (if one is required to perform the job in your state) should be checked. Finally, a preplacement examination will help determine the applicant's suitability for the position. All these factors have an impact on an employee's safety performance. However, equal employment opportunity must be maintained at all times. Always avoid discrimination on the basis of race, sex, age, or religion.

☐ Safety in Clinical Services

Clinical services are those departments or areas in the facility involved in patient care, including, for example, nursing, anesthesiology, and pathology. Such services encounter problems in patient care delivery that may not affect support services as much. Each service has its own unique hazards that distinguish it from other departments. Each of these individual risks should be dealt with directly through specific policies and procedures.

Although not all of the minute safety concerns of each clinical service can be described here, a few of the most common and prominent problems are highlighted.

Nursing

Two major sources of injury for nurses are back strain from lifting patients and cuts and punctures. Chapter 5 addresses proper lifting techniques. Nurses can avoid cuts and punctures by following these tips:

- Don't try to catch a falling object that is sharp or breakable.
- Don't force glass tubing. Use a lubricant and wear gloves.
- Dispose of syringes immediately after use and place them in a puncture-resistant container.
- Work slowly and carefully when inoculating a patient.

By far, the greatest number of cuts and punctures are needle-stick injuries. Although they are often a major problem in nursing, punctures from hypodermic needles may occur as often, or even more frequently, among housekeeping, laundry, and pathology personnel. Often, these incidents occur because of improper disposal of needles and sharps, such as when needles are carelessly discarded in plastic bags with other trash or are left on bedsheets where laundry personnel may inadvertently handle them.

In studies of this safety issue, researchers found that one of the reasons most frequently cited by nurses for needle sticks is unavailability of proper receptacles for used needles (Feldman, 1986, p. 15). Even when they were available, the receptacles were not emptied often enough and were usually full (see table 4-1 on p. 58). Nurses also recommended that these puncture-resistant receptacles be placed in every patient room, close to the bed. Another major cause of needle sticks is the recapping of used needles. Syringes should *never* be recapped, bent, broken, or cut after use.

Surgery, Special Care Units, and Dialysis

A primary concern in the surgery department and in dialysis and special care units is electrical safety. Sophisticated electrical equipment must be used here, with no margin for error. Here are some electrical safety measures:

- A system of preventive maintenance should be established whereby all electrical equipment is inspected regularly and constantly maintained to prevent hazards. The Joint Commission on Accreditation of Healthcare Organizations (Joint Commission) requires specific inspection programs for patient-use and non-patient-use equipment.
- Electrical cords should not be frayed or exposed.
- The maintenance or engineering department should maintain compliance with NFPA 101 (Life Safety Code for the National Fire Protection Association).
- Those using the equipment should visually inspect it before use.
- Those using the equipment must also receive orientation and at least annual continuing education on proper electrical safety.
- The emergency power generator must be reliable and adequate to provide electricity to crucial life support equipment during interruption of the normal electrical source.
- Dialysis machines should be maintained at the correct temperature range (35° to 40° C, 95° to 104° F) and conductivity (12 to 14 milliohms).
- Electrical cords should be secured and kept out of high-traffic areas to avoid tripping hazards.

Laser Safety

Laser is an acronym for Light Amplification by Stimulated Emission of Radiation. Lasers have recently come into wide use in medical surgery and are often considered preferable to the scalpel because they can eliminate extensive bleeding. Lasers have a wide variety of surgical uses, including gynecological, general, plastic, and eye surgeries. However, they can also generate dangerous nonionizing radiation, create hazards to vision, and give off smoke and fumes.

The health care facility should have a laser safety program outlined in policies and procedures and headed by a laser safety officer (LSO). The program should train and protect all potentially affected personnel, including staff nurses, operating room technicians, physicians, anesthesia staff, and laser support personnel. Laser safety guidelines include the following:

- The laser should be hooked up to its own transformer, emergency power, and a safety interlock.
- An approved fire extinguisher should be readily available in case of fire.
- All affected personnel and patients should wear appropriate eye protection.
- A sign on the door should warn of laser use and possible eye damage.
- A program of preventive maintenance for laser equipment should be in place.
- All personnel involved in the use of lasers should take part in a medical surveillance program to prevent eye damage.
- The smoke created during laser use can be irritating and dangerous and should be evacuated using a commercial smoke evacuator. The evacuated smoke should be filtered before it is exhausted from the building.

Anesthesiology

Special care should be taken to ensure the safe administration of anesthetic gases. Written safety regulations must be established to minimize electrical hazards. If flammable agents are used, all sources of ignition or explosion should be removed. In addition, personnel must be protected from excessive exposure to anesthetizing agents, which may cause adverse health effects. Effective gas-scavenging systems should be instituted, along with regularly scheduled maintenance of anesthesia equipment to prevent leakage.

Respiratory Therapy

Oxygen fires constitute the foremost threat in respiratory therapy. Signs must demarcate areas where oxygen is in use, and smoking must be prohibited in these areas. Electrical equipment that could generate sparks or raise the temperature substantially should be prohibited. Motorized beds used with oxygen tents should be approved by Underwriters Laboratories. Chapter 7 discusses the safe handling and storage of compressed gas cylinders (including oxygen).

Radiology and Nuclear Medicine

It is imperative for the radiology and nuclear medicine departments to have written policies and procedures for the safe use, storage, and disposal of radiological materials (based on Nuclear Regulatory Commission requirements) and for the protection of workers from ionizing radiation. Radiological materials vary in hazardousness, and their radioactive wastes may be disposed of in a variety of ways, depending on their type. Trained and knowledgeable personnel, with the help of the radiation safety committee, should establish procedures based on federal, state, and local rules.

X-ray machines emit dangerous radiation and must be used carefully. The reproductive systems of patients and technicians should be shielded and kept at a protective distance from the source of the radiation at all times. In addition, adequate protection should be provided for employees working around implant patients because implants may also give off potentially dangerous levels of radiation. Employees affected by radiation may include personnel from nursing, housekeeping, radiology, and pathology.

Pathology

All hazardous materials and wastes from the pathology department must be handled according to applicable regulations and guidelines (see chapter 6 for further discussion of hazardous materials management). Precautions against needle sticks and cuts as well as other basic safety measures should be observed. Figure 4-1 (see p. 53) summarizes pathology safety precautions.

Emergency

The emergency department is frequently the busiest department in the hospital. Patients and relatives are often in a distracted state, which can be exacerbated by long waits. Security must be adequate in emergency departments, and emergency staff should work to calm emergency room visitors. Staff members who may have contact with blood, including those who clean up spills of blood, must be adequately protected against blood-borne infectious diseases (as described later in this chapter).

Pharmacy

The pharmacy department plays an important role in patient treatment and so must be operated in a safe and organized manner. All drugs should be stored securely and under prescribed conditions for temperature, light, and other variables, and the pharmacist must fill all prescriptions. If an order is illegible, the pharmacist should contact the prescribing professional, thereby avoiding a large source of medication errors.

Drugs should be labeled with the patient's full name and room number. Stock should be inspected regularly, and outdated drugs should be disposed of properly. Often, outdated drugs can be returned to the supplier for credit. Cytotoxic drugs should be handled cautiously, according to relevant guidelines (see chapter 6 for a more extensive discussion of guidelines for the handling of chemotherapeutic agents). Figure 4-2 (see p. 54) shows a pharmacy safety checklist.

□ Safety for Support Services

Support services refers to those departments (such as housekeeping and dietary) or areas (such as offices) acting in a function that indirectly (but still measurably) contributes to patient care. At first glance, these functions may not seem to pose the overt hazards that trouble clinical services. However, offices are frequent sites for tripping and falls, some cleaning agents may threaten the health of housekeeping employees, and many of the tools and techniques used in the preparation of food can predispose food service employees to accidents.

Administrative Offices

Especially in administrative offices, electrical cords may cause employees to trip and fall. Use of extension cords should be avoided. All other exposed cords, whenever possible, should be taped to the floor. Anti-slip surfaces should be utilized for all uncarpeted floors, and stumbling hazards, such as frayed carpet and loose tiles, should be repaired. Adequate light must be provided.

The heating and air-conditioning system and vents should be inspected regularly with particular attention to symptoms of "sick building syndrome," a condition in which bacteria, dust, molds, and fumes are trapped in and continually circulated through the building. This condition may lead to chronic health problems, such as colds or other illnesses, among employees.

Safety guidelines for offices should consider these items:

- Sound electrical safety measures should be observed.
- Aisles should be wide enough and unobstructed to permit flow of personnel.
- Some duplicating machines use chemicals in toners and other fluids that could endanger employee health. Adequate ventilation should be provided around such equipment, and employees must be informed of the hazards and how to protect themselves (see the section on the "Hazard Communication Standard" in chapter 6).
- For sedentary or monotonous jobs such as data entry, ergonomic chairs should be provided and have casters that are designed for carpet or tile.

- If asbestos-containing material is present in wall insulation or floor or ceiling tiles, any activities that could disturb the material should be expressly forbidden, including puncturing, tearing, or ripping the materials or hanging pictures. Employees must be informed about the presence of the material and the ways to protect themselves.
- Nonsmokers should be protected from the smoke of smokers through mutually agreeable arrangements set forth in a written facilitywide smoking policy.

Housekeeping

In health care, an orderly, clean, and attractive facility is especially necessary. Indeed, in many areas strictly aseptic conditions must be maintained at all times. Housekeeping personnel must consequently be well trained in ensuring that these conditions exist. The importance of their role should be strongly emphasized. The following precautions should be observed by housekeeping employees:

- Training should encompass the safe use of electrical power equipment, especially electrical scrub machines and other cleaning equipment that will be used with or around water. (Figure 4-3 on p. 54 is a general list of equipment safety measures for all health care facility services.)
- Light bulbs should be changed carefully and not when the bulb is hot or when people are underneath the bulb being changed.
- Electrical equipment should be disconnected from the power source before it is cleaned.
- Cleaning agents proved to be toxic to human health, highly flammable, or explosive should be replaced whenever possible with less dangerous materials. Use of gasoline, benzene, and carbon tetrachloride should be prohibited. The use of aerosol spray cans should be limited; they can be an irritant to patients and employees.
- Employees must be informed about the hazardous chemicals they work with and be trained in their safe use.
- Containers of hazardous chemicals used in cleaning must be properly labeled with name, health effects, and protective measures, according to the Hazard Communication Standard labeling requirements.
- Housekeeping employees should be thoroughly trained in proper disposal of hazardous and infectious wastes. Many health care facilities treat hazardous and infectious waste handling as a separate job title and position that requires specific training and certain physical and intellectual abilities and is within the housekeeping, risk management, or safety department.
- Housekeeping staff or other employees responsible for cleanups must be trained in specific procedures for cleanup of hazardous, infectious, cytotoxic, and radioactive spills. These tasks may be done by personnel specifically knowledgeable about such cleanup procedures, such as the staff of the pathology, pharmacy, or nuclear medicine department.

Dietary

The preparation of food presents plentiful opportunities for accidents, injuries, and the spread of disease. Figure 4-4 (see p. 55) suggests protective clothing for dietary and other support services staff. The following guidelines are helpful in averting frequent dietary incidents:

- An experienced, knowledgeable, and well-trained individual should direct the department and ensure food service safety.
- Dietary employees should be trained in safe food preparation procedures.
- Personal hygiene is of the utmost concern. Clothing and hairstyles must be in accordance with federal and state regulations.
- Before they are hired, employees should undergo a medical examination, including a chest X ray and blood tests.
- Regular handwashing cannot be overemphasized and should be required of all dietary personnel.
- Pest control should be adequate. Pesticides should not be allowed to contaminate food, and only trained personnel should apply pesticides.
- Foods should be stored at adequate temperatures and not allowed to spoil. (Figure 4-5 on p. 56 lists general sanitation measures.)
- Floors must be promptly cleaned of spills, and employees should be required to wear shoes with nonskid soles to avoid slips and falls.
- Glass and china should be stored conveniently and safely.
- Workers should be trained in the safe handling of knives and other cutting equipment.
- For prevention of burns:
  - Potholders should be abundant and accessible.
  - Hot foods should be poured away from the body.
  - Handles of pots and pans should be turned away from the edge of the range.
  - Minor burns should be treated immediately by running cold water over them or applying ice.
- When washing dishes in a sink, employees should keep glassware separate from metal utensils and wash knives individually and carefully.

Engineering

Maintenance areas in health care facilities can pose a number of dangers to employees. Employees should be aware of the specific hazards in their work areas. The following are some general guidelines for maintenance areas:

- Blade guards must be installed on table saws, band saws, and radial arm saws. If saws are used for ripping, antikickback devices must be installed.
- All electrical equipment must be properly grounded or double-insulated.
- All extension cords must be of the three-wire type and of sufficient capacity to safely carry the current drawn by any device that is to be operated from the cord. Extension cords may be used only in temporary locations and may not be substituted for fixed wiring.
- Metal ladders must never be used by employees who are working on electrical equipment or wiring or who are changing light bulbs.
- Electrical switch lock-outs or tags must be used when repairs are being made on any machinery.
- Broken ladders must be destroyed or they must be tagged, removed from service, and repaired.
- Protective clothing and equipment must be provided for and worn by all employees exposed to hazards requiring protection, such as:
  - Gloves—for handling hot, wet, or sharp objects and chemicals
  - Hearing protection—for protection from noise
  - Eye and face protection—for protection from chips, sparks, glare, and splashes

- All gasoline-powered equipment must be properly maintained and only operated in well-ventilated areas to prevent the buildup of carbon monoxide.
- All hand tools must be kept in good repair and stored properly.
- Some laboratories use sodium azide in automatic blood-cell counting. When plumbing repair work is to be performed in laboratories where sodium azide is used, the pipes must first be decontaminated. A violent explosion can result if a buildup of sodium azide exists in the pipes. A copy of the decontamination procedure is available from the National Institute for Occupational Safety and Health.

Some more common health hazards found in maintenance areas include the following:

- *Asbestos* is often used as an insulating material for steam pipes in older buildings (see chapter 6 for more information on asbestos).
- *Carbon monoxide* is given off by gasoline-powered engines on auxiliary power generators.
- *Ammonia* may be used as a liquid cleaning agent or as a refrigerant gas.
- *Drain-cleaning chemicals* can damage the eyes and burn the skin.
- *Noise* exposure exceeding allowable limits often occurs in boiler rooms.
- *Paints and adhesives* contain a wide variety of solvents. These compounds should only be used in areas that are adequately ventilated.
- *Solvents* such as acetone may be used for cleaning parts in maintenance areas.
- *Pesticides* may be used throughout the facility for fumigation and extermination of pests.
- *Welding fumes* contain the fumes of the metals being joined and the filler material used, as well as the coating on the welding rods. Excessive exposures can occur when maintenance personnel weld in confined spaces.

Central Supply

Receiving, packaging, processing, and distribution operations occur in central supply. The major responsibility of the department focuses on materials handling.

These safety and health concerns are common in central supply:

- Cuts, bruises, and puncture wounds from blades, needles, knives, and broken glass often occur. Procedures for safe collection and disposal of hazardous instruments should be reviewed regularly. Employees should handle returned items based on the assumption that they contain sharp or hazardous instruments.
- Because strains, sprains, and back injuries also occur frequently in central supply areas, employees should be instructed in proper materials handling techniques.
- To prevent burns from steam and overexposure to ethylene oxide (EtO), sterilization equipment must be used properly. Effects from inhalation of EtO vapors include respiratory irritation and lung injury, headaches, nausea, and vomiting. Employers must be in compliance with the Occupational Safety and Health Administration's (OSHA's) ethylene oxide standard (29 C.F.R. 1910.1047), which includes a short-term exposure limit called an "excursion limit." Compliance with this standard includes:
  - — *Monitoring:* Performing initial monitoring to determine exposure.
  - — *Termination of monitoring:* Based on action level of initial monitoring.

- *Regulated areas:* Establishing and marking regulated areas and limiting them to authorized personnel.
- *Medical surveillance:* Instituting a medical surveillance program for all employees who are, or may be, exposed to EtO at or above the action level for at least 30 days a year, whether or not they use respirators.
- *Methods of compliance:* Implementing engineering and work practice controls to reduce and maintain employee exposure in accordance with the standard.
- *Compliance program:* Where exposure or excursion limit is exceeded, establishing a written program to reduce employee exposure to within acceptable limits. The program must include a schedule for periodic leak detection surveys and a written plan for emergency situations.
- *Respirators:* Providing respirators that comply with OSHA requirements.
- *Protective clothing and equipment:* Where eye or skin contact with liquid EtO or EtO solutions may occur, providing proper protective equipment and clothing at no cost to the employee.
- *Communication of hazards:* Posting and maintaining legible signs marking regulated areas and entrances to regulated areas, which includes labeling containers of EtO in certain situations. Labels must comply with requirements of the Hazard Communication Standard (see chapter 6).
- *Information and training:* Providing information and training on EtO at the time of initial assignment and at least annually thereafter.

• Chairs, boxes, and other objects inappropriately used for climbing are a common cause of falls. Step stools and ladders should be available for employees to reach high shelves in storage areas.

☐ Safety for Volunteers

Health care facilities are lucky in that they can draw on a resource most other businesses lack—volunteers. These can range from visiting choirs during the holidays to the regular, daily volunteer. Volunteers are usually people committed to the giving of themselves to help others, and their presence can have a favorable effect on patient morale.

Consequently, the facility has a corresponding responsibility to ensure a safe atmosphere and safety training for volunteers. Volunteers will need safety training for any tasks they are to perform, such as directing visitors and accompanying patients on walks through the facility and grounds. Daily volunteers should participate in fire and disaster preparedness training so that they can assist in the event of an emergency.

While on duty, all volunteers should wear ID badges and appropriate clothing, such as low-heeled shoes. Volunteers who are professionally qualified should have any license(s) their vocation requires. Separate policies and procedures should describe precautions for volunteers. Because the activities in which volunteers are involved can take them into virtually all facility areas, management and administration should take special care to protect their safety.

☐ Infection Control

Although a health care facility is a place where people go to get well, it is also a place where microorganisms may thrive and promote disease. Nosocomial (hospital-acquired) infections have long been a source of concern in health care. Measures to combat such infections, called infection control, are important to ensure successful patient outcomes and to protect all who pass through the doors of the facility from the risk of contracting disease.

The Joint Commission requires an infection control committee to bear the primary responsibility for control of nosocomial infections. The committee should include representation from the medical staff, administration, nursing, and, when available, the microbiology section of pathology. The housekeeping, laundry, central services, dietary, engineering/maintenance, and pharmacy departments must also provide representation, at least on a consultative basis. A liaison member from the safety committee may also participate, if desired.

Because the infection control committee is vested with this responsibility, infection control has not been considered an element in traditional safety. It is up to the safety director or safety committee, however, to assist in infection control and encourage staff members to utilize proper infection control methods. Training in proper infection control techniques should receive equal emphasis in the facility's staff education program. Safe practices and proper infection control measures intersect in nearly every area of health care facility operation—from the cleaning of patient areas to the careful inoculation of patients. Therefore, safety department personnel, along with clinical and support staff, should be educated about infection control.

Employees may not realize that the potential for infection exists through various means:

- *Airborne agents.* Bacteria and other pathogenic agents can become airborne through sneezing and coughing as well as through such avoidable accidents as spills and breakage of containers.
- *Ingestion.* Employees and patients can easily ingest infectious agents as they eat, drink, or smoke. This source of infection can be minimized through handwashing before all meals. (This includes patients, some of whom may have to be assisted in washing their hands.) Similarly, employees should only eat, drink, or smoke in designated lounges, not in work areas. They should be provided with a separate place to store their lunches, that is, not near nonfood substances such as medication, specimens, waste, solvents, or other chemicals.
- *Direct inoculation.* Needle sticks comprise nearly 20 percent of occupational injuries to nurses. Nurses may be careless, tired, or rushed, or patients may move suddenly or be uncooperative, and the nurse will then accidentally inoculate himself or herself. Needle sticks, or "hospital-acquired puncture conditions," as they are called, have the potential to spread such blood-borne infectious diseases as hepatitis B virus, syphilis, and AIDS.
- *Skin contact.* Pathogenic microorganisms can enter the body through the skin. Mucous membranes such as the eyes, nose, and mouth are particularly susceptible. Cuts or abrasions as small as a hangnail may provide a portal of entry for an infectious agent. Gloves and face masks are among the effective protection measures to prevent parenteral (mucous membrane) contact with infectious agents.

These basic facts of infection control should be explained to all employees, along with methods to avert transmission. Yet the simplest infection control procedure is often the most neglected—handwashing (after contact with an infected person, before meals, after using the restroom, after removing gloves, and after handling chemicals). Adequate lavatory facilities, with soap and towels, should be available to all staff members. There are many infection control techniques, most of which rest on a basis of safe, careful work habits.

☐ AIDS and Hepatitis B: Protection for Health Care Employees

Acquired immunodeficiency syndrome (AIDS) is a painful and tragic disease fraught with fear and ignorance. It is also a disease that continues to infect growing numbers. According to OSHA and the Centers for Disease Control (CDC), as many as 270,000 people will be sick with the disease in 1991, most of whom will die within a few months to a few years. Perhaps no other industry will be affected more than health care, and among the many issues AIDS raises for health care providers is how to protect employees. Throughout the country, AIDS has provoked an uproar among health care workers. Doctors have refused to treat AIDS patients, nurses have sued for lack of training in how to protect themselves as they care for victims of the disease, and OSHA has cited facilities for failure to establish precautions.

Along with awareness of AIDS, there has been a resurgence of interest in hepatitis B virus (HBV), a serious blood-borne infectious disease that attacks and inflames the liver. According to the CDC, HBV is the major infectious occupational health hazard in the health care industry. Approximately 18,000 health care workers contract HBV each year, and as many as 300 a year die from complications related to the disease.

Regulatory Control

The Occupational Safety and Health Administration and the Department of Health and Human Services (HHS) have published recommendations for protection of health care workers from AIDS, HBV, and other blood-borne infection hazards (see the *Federal Register*, May 30, 1989). Furthermore, OSHA will enforce these regulations through an inspection and citation process. Between 150 and 200 unannounced inspections were to have taken place in 1989. Moreover, OSHA intends to publish a standard on this topic with the force of law by 1991. The major recommendations currently center on education, protective procedures, and training.

Education

All employees should receive basic AIDS/HBV education, including information about the various means of transmission. The primary means of transmission for AIDS is sexual. There is no evidence that either HBV or the AIDS virus can be transmitted through casual contact, airborne routes, or contaminated food or drinking water. Workers may be exposed to the viruses through parenteral contact with infected body fluids or tissues. The viruses have been isolated in blood, semen, amniotic fluid, saliva, tears, urine, vaginal secretions, cerebrospinal fluid, and possibly human breast milk. However, because of the minute levels of the virus present in all these fluids except blood, infection through contact with these fluids is less likely. By far, the fluid most likely to transmit the viruses through occupational exposure is blood.

The occupational risk of contracting HBV is much higher than that for AIDS. Infections following puncture by an infected needle range from 6 percent to 30 percent for HBV, compared to less than 1 percent for AIDS. Despite this,

AIDS deserves the attention of facility administration. Employee fear of AIDS can lead to litigation by patients who were refused care and employees who were exposed to the virus during their work. In addition, regulatory agencies can cite the facility for failure to provide a safe atmosphere, and employee unions may become involved.

Protective Procedures

In order to provide the highest level of protection for personnel, OSHA divides health care tasks into three categories, each requiring a different degree of protection. (The following are the most current guidelines as this book goes to press. Specific categories and requirements are subject to change, so the reader should consult the latest guidelines and standards.)

- *Category I.* This category encompasses tasks that involve exposure to blood, body fluids, or tissues as a normal condition of the employee's job description. This includes tasks with a potential for mucous membrane contact with these fluids and tissues or a possibility of spills or splashes of them. Examples of Category I tasks are surgery and drawing blood. Employees who engage in Category I tasks should be required to use personal protective equipment such as surgical latex gloves, gowns, masks, and eye protectors, depending on the work. Employees must be trained in the proper use of this equipment.
- *Category II.* This class comprises tasks with no exposure to blood, body fluids, or tissues as a normal condition of the employee's job description but that may require unplanned Category I tasks. For example, some activities required by police and paramedic work may involve splashing blood or profuse bleeding. Category II personnel must be provided ready access to personal protective equipment. For instance, paramedics should have latex gloves, face masks, eye protection, gowns, and protective resuscitation devices close at hand in the ambulance. Again, personnel must be trained in the use of this equipment.
- *Category III.* Category III tasks involve no foreseeable exposure to infectious body fluids as a normal condition of the employee's job description. This classification applies to employees not expected as part of their employment to perform or assist in medical care. Examples include dietary and office personnel. Those in Category III jobs need not have ready access to personal protective equipment but should still receive basic education on AIDS and other blood-borne diseases.

Universal Precautions

In addition to the protection of employees through the categorization of tasks, the facility should implement policies regarding the handling of patient waste. The Centers for Disease Control has encouraged facilities to adopt a guarded waste-handling philosophy by introducing the concept of "universal precautions." Universal precautions refers to the assumption that all body fluids or tissues are potentially infectious.

This has been interpreted to mean that all patient-contact waste should be handled as infectious. Although the CDC has indicated that this extreme measure may not have been its intent, universal precautions should serve as a motivator for facilities to treat patient-contact waste cautiously and with attention to the protection of employees, patients, and the community. This careful approach reinforces the facility's other blood-borne infectious disease procedures.

Training

Besides education on the fundamentals of AIDS and HBV, employees must also be trained to work safely with or around AIDS patients. In particular, OSHA's most recent classification system for health care tasks should be explained, along with the protective measures for each category. Employees in each category must be trained in the protective measures for those tasks.

In addition, the training should specify the locations of personal protective equipment and explain how to decontaminate or dispose of it after use. It should also be stressed that the protective equipment is not invulnerable, especially when used carelessly or inconsistently. Adequate protection from blood-borne infectious disease relies heavily on the safe work habits and infection control procedures of employees, including handwashing (even when gloves are used). Finally, housekeeping employees and other employees should be trained in spill cleanup and in what to do in the event of exposure to body fluids. Figure 4-6 (see p. 57) presents 12 questions that can be used as a checklist in training employees to protect themselves from AIDS and other blood-borne infectious diseases.

The facility should write policies and procedures for AIDS protection with attention to the three categories of tasks. Perhaps just as important as training and the implementation of protective measures, administrators must respond to employee fears. Employees who detect sincere concern on the part of the administration are more likely to take an active role in protecting themselves. Again, because this area of liability and responsibility is relatively new, standards and guidelines change rapidly. Consequently, health care administrators and personnel are urged to stay abreast of the most recent requirements.

□ Helicopter Safety

Transportation of the sick and injured by air predates even the airplane. In 1870, during the Franco-Prussian War, injured French soldiers were evacuated from battlefields by hot-air balloons. Airlifts during World War II saved thousands of lives, and beginning with the Korean War, helicopters boosted the success of medical air evacuation. In the mid-1960s, hospitals began to employ helicopters for patient transport, and today there are over 150 emergency medical helicopter programs in the United States.

In order to set up a program, some research into the services available in your area and the safety records of the organizations offering such services will be necessary. The American Society of Hospital-Based Emergency Air Medical Services (ASHBEAMS) sets standards for the quality of patient care and the safety of operation of its more than 150 member programs. The organization can provide information on the availability and quality of helicopter programs in your area.

Once the services of a medical air transport company have been contracted, the facility must prepare a landing pad that meets Federal Aviation Authority (FAA) requirements. The authority having jurisdiction over the landing and use of medical air transport, which may be the fire or police department or another department, should be contacted for restrictions on the location of this site. A rooftop landing pad may not always be the best choice because of the difficulties it may present for fire, police, or other personnel to reach the pad if they need to become involved.

During a disaster or other emergency, or if a regular landing pad is not established, it may be necessary to set up a field landing site. A plan should address what type of place will be used in this situation; a playground, open field, or parking lot is best. Personnel involved in this landing must have expertise in medical air evacuation and helicopter site procedures. Many factors, such as mountainous or rough terrain, winds, bodies of water, and thermal currents, can affect the size and type of landing zone required.

The field site should meet basic FAA safety requirements. When a helicopter has been called to an emergency field site, all major obstructions should be removed and flares should be set up to mark the zone. Lights or flares should also designate the presence of poles, wires, power lines, or signs that the pilot may have difficulty seeing. The landing area should ideally be 100 feet by 100 feet or larger but may be a minimum of 75 feet by 75 feet.

Some general helicopter safety precautions should be observed:

1. Wait for the pilot to motion you to the helicopter.
2. Always approach a helicopter from the front, walking in a crouched position.
3. When a helicopter lands on a slope, approach it from the downhill side rather than the uphill side.
4. Never approach the area of the tail rotor.
5. Allow only authorized personnel within 100 feet of the aircraft.
6. Smoking should be prohibited within 100 feet of the helicopter.
7. Only the flight crew should open and close helicopter doors and secure patients and equipment.

When the facility establishes or contracts an air medical transport service, it must develop policies and procedures to protect the safety of patients and ground personnel.

□ Conclusion

To ensure safe and healthful working conditions in a health care facility, it is essential to implement individualized departmental safety practices. These must be described in specific policies and procedures that are regularly reviewed and updated. The specific procedures then fit into the comprehensive safety management program, as department-specific and facilitywide risks are coordinated through a systematic approach to safety.

Figure 4-1. Laboratory Safety Precautions

- Permit only authorized personnel in the laboratory. Designate areas for other staff and for patients.
- Observe all signs denoting hazardous areas where there are infectious agents and toxic substances.
- Walk carefully. Floors in lab areas where paraffin is used are extremely slippery.
- Before and after work and if a spill occurs, wash all countertops with a 1:500 dilution of a suitable disinfectant to destroy bacteria or with 1 percent chlorine bleach to destroy viruses.
- Wash hands often with disinfectant soap, and always wash before leaving the work area.
- Cleanse and dress a cut or puncture immediately, noting the cause of injury and the material handled.
- Report any injury. If a possibility exists of exposure to infection, seek medical attention.
- Treat all organisms as pathogens. Do not remove infectious materials from specified areas.
- Handle all tissue samples, bloods, and serums as though they were from infected patients. Dispose of clots in disinfectant-soaked towels. Thoroughly disinfect all tubes, needles, and syringes.
- Use all necessary personal protective equipment (such as a face mask and surgical latex or other appropriate gloves) when handling infectious materials.
- Wash hands thoroughly after handling hazardous or infectious materials, even if gloves were worn.
- Identify highly infectious agents during use and prior to storage with a label on the container. Identify incubator trays or racks containing hazardous materials.
- Put all hazardous material in labeled plastic bags or other appropriate container for disposal.
- Use both hands when handling large bottles and never lift them by the top alone.
- File an ampule at the demarcation prior to removing the tip, and cover the top with gauze.
- Use a mechanical pipette aid to draw material into a pipette. Do not ever use your mouth to suck any material into a pipette.
- Without splashing, place used pipettes carefully, tip down, into a 1:500 dilution of a suitable disinfectant or 3 percent phenol for 24 hours before washing or disposing of them. Plug all pipettes with cotton.
- Never place pipettes or hot wire loops in culture fluid.
- Remove all broken glass from countertops to prevent slivers from cutting hands, arms, and elbows.
- Discard all glassware, syringes, and needles into labeled, puncture-resistant containers for this purpose. Disinfect such items if necessary.
- Place petri dishes containing infected cultures first in a closed container and then in an open bag with an airtight seal. Autoclave the bag and contents at the usual temperature and pressure for at least 45 minutes or the required time. After autoclaving, seal the bag and dispose of it.
- Wear gloves to remove materials from ovens and autoclaves.
- Observe usage rules on all laminar flow hoods.
- Chain gas cylinders in place. If empty, label them. Separate full cylinders from empty ones. When removing them, use a dolly.
- Ensure that hazardous chemicals are appropriately labeled at all times.
- Use only self-adhesive labels.
- Never remove materials and equipment from one laboratory to another laboratory without permission.

Figure 4-2. Pharmacy Safety Checklist

- Is the pharmaceutical service directed by a professionally competent and legally qualified pharmacist and staffed by a sufficient number of competent personnel?
- Do nonpharmacist personnel work under the direct supervision of a licensed pharmacist?
- Are drugs stored under proper conditions of sanitation, temperature, light, moisture, ventilation, segregation, and security?
  — Are biologicals and other thermolabile medications stored in a separate compartment within a refrigerator that is capable of maintaining the necessary temperature?
  — Are drugs for external use stored separately from oral and injectable medications?
- Does the director of pharmacy conduct at least monthly inspections of all nursing care units or other areas of the facility where medications are dispensed, administered, and stored? Are outdated drugs identified and their distribution and administration prevented?
- Is the distribution and administration of controlled drugs documented?
- Is the metric system and the unit dose drug distribution system used for all medications?
- Are metric/apothecaries' weight and measure conversion charts available to those who may require them?
- Is a Class II Type A or B biological safety cabinet used for mixing chemotherapeutic drugs?
- Is authoritative, current antidote information and the telephone number of the regional poison-control center readily available in the pharmacy for emergency reference?
- Are all drugs, chemicals, and biologicals clearly and accurately labeled? All prescriptions should be labeled with the following:
  — Name, address, and telephone number of the facility pharmacy
  — Date
  — Prescription serial number
  — Full name of patient
  — Name of the drug; strength and amount dispensed
  — Directions for patient use
  — Name or initials of prescribing practitioner
  — Initials of the dispensing individual
  — Any required Drug Enforcement Administration cautionary label on controlled substance drugs
  — Any other pertinent cautionary labels
- Are pharmacy personnel adequately trained for all the tasks they will perform?
- Does the pharmacy conduct a drug monitoring program for patients that reviews patients' drug regimens for any potential interactions, interferences, or incompatibilities?
- Does the director of pharmacy regularly participate in the education of medical and nursing staff regarding the use of drugs and biologicals in the facility?
- Do written policies and procedures regulate all pharmacy practices?

Figure 4-3. General Equipment Safety Measures

- Read the instructions that accompany a new piece of equipment before using it.
- Carry portable equipment such as a mop or broom close to the body to avoid injuring anyone.
- Station equipment out of the way. Never permit it to block exits, fire doors, fire extinguisher or fire hose cabinets, stairwells, or elevators.
- Clean equipment after use. Turn buckets upside down to dry thoroughly. Mops and cleaning cloths should be changed with each shift.
- Keep equipment in good repair: nuts and bolts tight, broken parts repaired or replaced.
- Report broken equipment immediately, remove it from service, and label the equipment as defective until repaired. Do not put broken equipment in a storage area containing operable equipment.
- Make sure electrical equipment is in working order and is grounded when in use. Do not use adapters. When using electrical rotary cleaning machines on wet floors, make sure all wiring and connections are sound.
- Wear rubber-soled shoes or rubber slipovers to prevent slipping.
- Do not clean ramps with power equipment.
- Make sure an adequate number of various sizes and types of ladders are available and in good repair. Set ladders firmly in position, and never stand on the top two rungs or steps. Do not use chairs, tables, or other furniture as stools or ladders.

Figure 4-4. Protective Clothing for Support Services Personnel

Central Service

- Impervious gloves to eliminate skin contact with irritating chemicals.
- Respirator—used by people who are trained and in a medical surveillance/training program for respirator use.
- Chemical apron and full-face shield, when required.

Dietary

- Low-heeled shoes with slip-resistant soles and boots for wet areas.
- Impervious gloves for washing pots and pans and for consistently wet hands.
- Metal mesh gloves for meatcutters and others who use knives frequently.
- Rubber gloves and goggles or a face shield for handlers of concentrated liquid ammonia, drain cleaners, strong caustic solutions for cleaning reusable filters, and oven cleaners.
- Disposable masks for persons sensitive to powdered soap or detergent dust.
- Hair nets in food preparation and serving areas to minimize contamination of food.

Housekeeping

- Heavy rubber aprons and impervious gloves for persons engaged primarily in removal of nonhazardous trash.
- Protective gloves for users of soaps, detergents, or solvents.
- Appropriate gloves and face/eye protection when handling hazardous or infectious waste. The Material Safety Data Sheet (MSDS) for the hazardous chemical being handled will specify appropriate personal protective equipment.
- Nonskid shoes or boots for persons who flush, strip, rinse, and wax floors.

Laboratories

- Chemical goggles or face shields for protection from splashes.
- Chemical-cartridge respirators for persons cleaning up spills or using large amounts of acid, bases, and so forth.
- Coats or aprons, which are removed when wearers leave the laboratory.
- All other personal protective equipment specified in MSDSs or required for protection from infection, such as appropriate gloves or a face mask or apron.

Laundry

- Protective clothing and masks for sorting contaminated linen.
- Appropriate gloves for handling potentially infectious linen.
- Gloves, aprons, and safety glasses for persons using bleaches and soaps.
- Hair nets to minimize contamination of clean linen.

Figure 4-5. General Sanitation Measures for Food Service

1. Keep all foods at safe temperatures. Bacteria grow best within the range of 50° to 140° F. Once food is prepared it should never be allowed to remain within that temperature range. All foods ready to be served should be kept at hot (above 140° F) or cold (below 45° F) temperatures.
   Cooked foods should be brought to a temperature above the bacteria-killing level and should be maintained at that temperature until they are served. Cold foods should be kept cold until they are served.
   Defrosting should be done far enough in advance so that it can be done in a refrigerator below 45° F.
2. Follow safe techniques for cooling or reheating leftovers. Cool all leftover hot foods quickly by placing them in shallow containers in the coolest area of the refrigerator. Reheat leftovers only once, bringing them above the 140° F killing point.
3. Avoid cross-contamination. If raw and ready-to-serve foods are mixed in processing or storage, bacteria from the raw foods may contaminate the ready-to-serve foods. Do not mix these foods, because they usually cannot be heated above killing temperature.
   Cross-contamination can also occur when cutting boards, knives, and appliances are not cleaned after use and are used for both types of food. These tools should be washed following each use.
4. Store food properly. Refrigerated foods should be covered to avoid contamination brought about by foods touching each other or the shelves and walls of the refrigerator. Sanitary storage temperatures for foods are:
   a. Dry—50-70° F
   b. Chilled—45° F or less
   c. Frozen—0° F or less
5. Handle food properly. Utensils or tools should be used to handle food rather than bare hands. If food must be touched, disposable plastic gloves must be worn. Never put a tasting spoon back into the food after it has been used.
6. Clean tableware, equipment, and utensils at appropriate temperatures. Mechanical dishwasher water should remain above the bacteria-killing point of 140° F with the final rinse temperature set at 180° F. Follow the manufacturer's instructions for positioning the dishes in the dishwasher. Use the appropriate detergent in the proper amount for both mechanical and hand washing. Rinse the dishwasher and clean the foodtraps following each meal. All appliances should be cleaned, sanitized, and protected against contamination.
7. Insist on good personal hygiene. Personnel must wash before beginning work, after using the restroom, and after touching any soiled item. To encourage these habits, handsoap and towels must be readily available in the kitchen and bathrooms. Bathrooms should also be kept very clean. Clean uniforms, hairnets, disposable plastic gloves, and personal protective equipment should be provided and used.
8. Have a liberal sick leave policy. Employees with sore throats, gastrointestinal infections, infected cuts, nasal discharge, burns, sores, or boils should be sent home or given other tasks to avoid infecting the entire facility.
9. Control insects and pests. Flies may transmit up to 30 types of bacteria, including those causing typhoid, dysentery, and diarrhea. Screens in windows and doors will help keep them out, but the best control is to eliminate their breeding ground. Keep all garbage cans covered, and promptly clean up all filth and debris in and around the facility.
   Roaches are another common pest. They are attracted to dark, damp, and dirty areas, such as near sinks, around water pipes, and in corners and crevices. They carry many bacteria, including salmonella. To control roach infestation, fill all cracks and crevices, keep all food service areas clean and orderly, and inspect all incoming supplies for signs of roaches.
   Rodents are the carriers of many dangerous bacteria and, due to their size, they can destroy much food. Cracks and crevices should be filled in and around the building to keep them out. Rodenticides also help control them. Good housekeeping methods and sanitary handling and storage are a primary defense against pests. Also, consult with a pest-control service.
10. Store chemical compounds away from foods. Always be certain that cleaning and disinfectant supplies are stored in distinctive containers that are clearly marked with contents, cautions, and first-aid measures. Keep all chemicals and cleaning solutions away from bulk storage areas.

Source: Reprinted, with permission, from National Safety Council. *Long Term Care Safety Management Manual: A Handbook for Practical Application.* Chicago: National Safety Council, 1987, pp. 36–38.

Figure 4-6. OSHA-Recommended Checklist for Employee Protection from HBV and HIV

1. Has a training and information program been established for employees actually or potentially exposed to blood or body fluids?
2. How often is training provided and does it cover:
   a. Universal precautions?
   b. Personal protective equipment?
   c. Workplace practices including blood drawing, room cleaning, laundry handling, cleanup of blood spills?
   d. Needle-stick exposure/management?
   e. Hepatitis B vaccination?
3. Does new employee orientation cover infectious disease control?
4. Does the employer evaluate the effectiveness of the training program through monitoring of employee compliance with the guidelines?
5. Have employees been informed of the precautionary measures outlined in the CDC guidelines?
6. Is personal protective equipment provided to employees? In all appropriate locations? (Specifically, are there gloves, masks, eye protection, gowns, as appropriate?)
7. Is the necessary equipment (mouthpieces, resuscitation bags, or other ventilation devices) provided for administering mouth-to-mouth resuscitation to potentially infected patients?
8. Does training identify the specific procedures implemented by the facility to provide protection, such as proper use of personal protective equipment?
9. Are equipment and materials available to comply with workplace practices, such as handwashing sinks, needle containers, detergents and disinfectants to clean up spills?
10. Are employees aware of specific workplace practices to follow when appropriate? Are the following emphasized:
    - Handwashing?
    - Handling sharp instruments?
    - Routine examinations?
    - Blood spills?
    - Handling of laundry?
    - Disposal of contaminated materials?
    - Reusable equipment?
11. Are workers aware of procedures to follow after needle sticks or blood exposure?
12. Is there a hepatitis B vaccination program? Do employees take advantage of it?

Table 4-1. Nurses' Ratings of Solutions to Reduce Needle Injuries

Solution	Rating (7-point scale; 7 is extremely effective)
1. Make more inspections of disposal units.	5.7
2. Have more disposal units emptied more often.	5.6
3. Make more needle disposal units available on the floor.	4.8
4. Use medication carts with disposal units on the cart.	4.3
5. Group discussions and peer interactions on methods to maintain safe stations and reduce injuries.	4.1
6. Have a needle disposal unit built into the wall of each patient's room.	3.9
7. Rewards and incentives to nursing stations with good safety records.	3.4
8. Increased use of safety posters, bulletin board notices, newsletters, and pamphlets on reducing needle injuries.	3.4
9. Rewards, incentives, and praise to individual nurses with good safety records.	3.3
10. More talks, information, and in-service classes on preventing needle injuries.	3.2

Source: Reprinted, with permission, from Feldman, R. H. L. Hospital injuries. *Occupational Health and Safety* 55(9):15, Sept. 1986.

Chapter 5
Patient Safety

During the course of any given patient's care, numerous opportunities present themselves for accidents and injuries. Many factors conspire to jeopardize patient safety. Patients may be confused, senile, weak, or agitated and may do things they would not do under ordinary circumstances. They may overestimate their ability to stand, walk, or perform other normally routine activities, or they may be dissatisfied with their care and treatment and lash out at facility personnel.

These conditions and others too countless to mention predispose patients to injuries sustained through slips, falls, burns, and fire and through patient care procedures such as being lifted and transported from one area of the facility to another. All of these incidents constitute "potentially compensable events"—occurrences over which patients may file claims and recover damages.

Any unsafe condition that affects patients will necessarily endanger employee well-being. Employee safety and patient safety converge in nearly every patient care activity and in many tasks not directly related to patient care. During patient lifting, for example, not only could the patient fall or twist a limb, but the attendant doing the lifting could strain or sprain his or her back or leg or arm muscles. An unmarked wet floor could cause a patient, employee, volunteer, or visitor to fall. Through attention to patient safety, then, the facility will accomplish several important objectives: reduce accidents and potentially compensable events among both employees and patients, enhance overall safety in the facility, and improve patient care.

□ Patient Relations

As any nurse knows, not all patients who have been injured "iatrogenically," or during patient care, file a malpractice claim or even a formal complaint. Yet others with less serious contentions sometimes do. What accounts for this inconsistency? Often, less tangible variables, such as the dissatisfaction of the patient or patient's family or feelings of depersonalization, may significantly influence a decision to take action against the facility. These feelings of dissatisfaction or depersonalization may even play a substantial role in the actual occurrence of patient accidents.

A major reason for patient dissatisfaction stems from the increasingly impersonal health care environment. Patients' desires for interaction, communication, and respect—all basic human needs—are often not being met during the course of treatment. Compounding this situation is that patients and their families often feel they have no avenue through which to express their concerns.

For both practical and humanitarian reasons, more health care facilities should enhance patient communication. Physicians must be encouraged to spend more time with patients and be open to questions or concerns. Nurses and attendants should be shown ways to improve their active listening skills.

In addition, a formal mechanism should exist whereby patient complaints are acknowledged and acted upon. The facility should develop a policy explaining patient rights and responsibilities and go over these with patients. There are multiple and diverse methods to better patient relations and, by extension, patient care. For example, figure 5-1 (see p. 68) illustrates a patient evaluation form that assesses the patient's satisfaction with care received. The facility is limited only by the creativity and empathy of its management and staff.

□ Using Restraints

Occasionally during their stay at a health care facility, patients will need to be restrained to prevent injury to themselves or others. Restraining a patient may be one of the most difficult decisions for a health care provider to make. The restraint may seem inhumane, yet the alternative of allowing patients to injure themselves or others may be equally inconsiderate.

One way to alleviate this source of concern is to train patient care staff—nurses, aides, physicians—in ways to discourage aggression. Health care personnel should understand that patients may be confused and apprehensive and that their personalities may be altered by medication or other treatment. This empathy with the patient's position will help staff realize that the patient's aggressive behavior is not a personal attack.

Health care employees should be instructed to approach angry patients with caution and sympathy. They should know how to talk in a soothing manner and ask about the problem without appearing confrontational. Again, employees should understand that good patient relations throughout the patient's stay can minimize the likelihood of aggressive behavior.

Invariably, some patients will require restraint. In addition to combative patients, senile individuals and those under the influence of medication or alcohol may need restraints. The decision to restrain should be in response to a specific event that demonstrates the danger the patient presents. Patients should never be restrained as a way to prevent or punish violent behavior or just because they *sometimes* show signs of dementia or aggression. An exception to this is patients who have a consistent record of sudden violence or of falls from bed or from a wheelchair. If all other efforts to correct this condition have failed, soft restraints used regularly are acceptable. The facility should be prepared to demonstrate a compelling reason for the use of restraints, and all proper authorization should be received.

The facility should implement a policy and procedure that specifies when restraint is appropriate, who should approve the decision, what means should be used to restrain, the maximum time a patient should be restrained, where the patient will be restrained, and the frequency of checks. The procedure on restraint should include these directions:

- Only use restraint as a last resort, but do not hesitate to use it when there is a clear and present danger to the patient, other patients, or staff. Document the provoking event on the chart.
- Remove the patient from populated areas before restraining.
- Explain to the patient what is being done and why. Encourage open discussion where this is possible.
- Search the patient for matches or cigarettes before removing or restraining him or her. These could be used in an attempt to get free of the restraints by burning them off.
- Never restrain or transport an unwilling patient alone.
- Have the attending physician or physician on call countersign the order to restrain.
- Only use bed restraints that are padded.
- Regularly check the patient for discomfort, chafing, tightness, and so forth. Document the checks in the chart.
- Ensure that the restraints do not limit circulation or choke or scratch patients.
- Never exceed prescribed time limits for physical restraint.

If a restraint is used in response to an event, those involved must record in an incident report what happened and the restraining measures that were used. Documentation that efforts were made to subdue the patient, that authorization was obtained, and that regular checks were made must be adequately explained in the report. The report will then serve as protection against liability and as a guide for what can be done better if such a situation should recur. Figure 5-2 (see p. 69) outlines a four-step approach to patient restraint.

□ Using Call Systems

Call systems can act as a tool for safety, but too often they become a source of irritation and tension between nurse and patient. To promote legitimate use of call systems, as well as adequate response, both patients and nurses need to be educated. Nurses must know that call systems are designed to encourage patients not to do things for which they need help, such as climbing over bedrails or grabbing for an item out of reach. Even though a call for help may seem to be a nuisance, nurses should be encouraged to consider what might happen if the patient attempts a potentially dangerous activity without assistance.

The nurse should explain to the patient the proper use of the call system. He or she should specify what the patient can do and should not attempt to do without assistance. Although nurses have many other duties, responding promptly and courteously to patient calls will encourage patients to use the system rather than attempt a dangerous activity. Call buttons should be placed within easy reach of patients' beds. (Some facilities attach the button to the patient's pillow, taking care that the patient does not become entangled in the cord.) Ensuring that call buttons are as close as possible to patients prevents a major falling hazard when patients attempt to use a button that is out of reach.

☐ Lifting and Transporting Patients

Back injuries and muscle strain from lifting patients represent, by most measures, the single greatest class of injuries to health care workers, especially nurses, orderlies, and nurses' aides. Some studies even report a greater incidence of lower-back injuries and pain among health care employees than among manual workers in industry. Much industrial lifting has all but been eliminated through automation, whereas health care personnel must still lift patients to help them stand, transfer them to a chair or wheelchair, or move them to a gurney. Moreover, patients can also be severely injured in lifting accidents.

Despite the seeming difficulty of the task, safe lifting of patients is possible. In fact, most injuries result from improper lifting techniques. It is essential that all personnel involved in lifting patients receive training on lifting techniques. Employee back injuries and patient fractures and contusions can be very serious, leading to pain, liability, costly workers' compensation claims, and lost work time. Providing adequate training and implementing safe practices can minimize this major risk to employees, patients, and the facility.

When transferring patients to a chair or wheelchair, follow these steps:

1. First sum up the situation and plan the lift.
2. Ask for help when you think the job may be too much for you. Establish a patient weight and mobility policy that mandates getting help or using a mechanical device before the patient is lifted.
3. Explain to the patient that he or she is to be moved and how.
4. Position the wheelchair parallel to the bed and lock both the bed casters and the wheelchair wheels.
5. Loosen bedclothes for easier motion.
6. Slide the patient, by pushing or pulling, as far as possible.
7. Ask the patient to flex his or her knees, if possible.
8. Place one arm under the patient's knees and the other under the far shoulder.
9. Help the patient to a seated position with feet on the floor.
10. Stand with feet slightly apart for good balance. Bend at the knees and hips.
11. Ask the patient to clasp arms around your neck, if possible.
12. Hold the patient close. Straighten legs to lift, pushing with thigh muscles.
13. Shift foot position to turn. DO NOT twist the torso.
14. Maintaining a hold on the patient, lower him or her into the chair.

Steps one through eight can also be used to help a patient sit up in bed. Instead of allowing the patient's feet to hang over the edge, however, the patient's upper body will be moved to a vertical position against the headboard, with legs extended on the bed.

In most cases in which a patient's entire body must be lifted, three people should participate. One grasps the head and shoulders, one the midsection, and the third holds the legs. All on the same side and in unison, they roll the patient onto his or her side so that their arms cradle the section each holds. They lift, again in unison, and turn to place the patient on the gurney or stretcher.

Some aids to lifting are available, such as the turning sheet and mechanical lifting devices. In using a turning sheet, one attendant stands on each side of the patient. The attendants hold the sheet at the patient's shoulders and buttocks, pull the sheet tight, and move the patient across the bed.

Mechanical lifting devices may be used in lifting particularly large or unresponsive patients. However, some evidence indicates that some devices may actually increase the work load and stress on the spine. Moreover, employees must be trained in the safe use of such devices and their limitations. The manufacturer's instructions must always be carefully followed.

☐ Preventing Slips and Falls

Studies consistently show that falls represent the single greatest cause of injury to patients during their stay at a health care facility. Indeed, much research suggests that up to 70 or 80 percent of patient accidents involve falls, a figure that may actually be greater for residents in a nursing home (Rusting, 1985, pp. 5–8). Risk factors may differ widely from facility to facility, but characteristics often correlated with frequent falls are age (those over 65 are more likely to fall), mental disturbance (including temporary agitation in those otherwise stable), weakened physical condition, and the taking of psychoactive drugs or a combination of medications.

Research also indicates that the great majority of falls occur in patient rooms, most either within feet of the bed or en route to the private bathroom. However, falls are in no way limited to these areas or to individuals displaying these specific risk factors. Every facility must assess those at risk within its own walls and respond to identified hazards through a system of prevention.

By far, the single most effective control measure is basic housekeeping. Often, simple spills or obstructions on the floor are the cause of falls; for example, water, food, and urine are frequent culprits. By removing spills immediately, staff members will eliminate a major source of costly and potentially debilitating falls. Spills can be prevented by delivering water in glasses on trays rather than in individual pitchers that often spill on the floor, by monitoring patients or residents who suffer from incontinence, and by reminding dietary personnel to carry food more carefully and slowly.

It is important to know your patients. Nurses and other attendants should be constantly aware of any conditions that patients display, whether temporary or permanent, that could predispose them to falls. This is particularly important in a long-term care setting, where patterns of behavior become evident. However, risk of falls in acute care facilities may be more insidious because patients who would not normally be considered at risk may temporarily be in a condition that promotes falling.

Some facilities have instituted programs that assess all patients on admittance as to their likelihood of falling. Factors such as a history of having fallen at home, poor eyesight, an unsteady gait, combination prescriptions, preoperative or postoperative conditions, and an uncooperative or belligerent attitude can all be assessed to determine the degree of risk. Those likely to fall are identified through some marking, such as red tape on their identification bracelets or kardex. Attendants are trained to keep a sharp eye on these individuals, and the list is updated throughout the day. Figure 5-3 (see p. 70) shows a sample daily fall-prevention list, which should be kept in the nursing unit.

In addition to a formal program of patient fall prevention, attendants should know basic fall-prevention measures:

1. Keep patient belongings and call buttons close to the bed so that patients do not have to reach too far for them, thus avoiding slipping and falling. Place call buttons within reach in the bathroom, close to the commode and shower.

2. Respond to trends in falls with new programs and patient fall-prevention in-service education.
3. Keep lighting bright in corridors and public areas.
4. Encourage patients to go to the bathroom before they go to bed. Even this simple measure can reduce nighttime falls.
5. Reevaluate drug treatment that contributes to frequent falls and constant disorientation.
6. Where possible, help nursing home residents to correct physical disabilities through physical therapy and walking aids.
7. Increase nursing coverage during high-risk activities such as getting out of bed and going to the bathroom.
8. Work to subdue hostile patients. Anger and resentment have been shown to contribute to falls.
9. Introduce softer surfaces for floors or furniture, and provide grab bars and handrails throughout the facility.
10. Use safety devices such as nonslip surfaces and footstools with rubber feet.
11. Use bedrails.
12. Repair torn carpet, and remove other obstructions from patient areas.

Through staff involvement and a philosophy of prevention, the facility can significantly reduce dangerous and costly patient falls.

☐ Preventing Burns

Although the incidence of burns in health care facilities is lower than the number of falls, burns can still inflict considerable pain and prolong patient stays. Burns are represented to an inordinate degree in neglect and malpractice suits, particularly in long-term care, where residents' ability to protect themselves from scalding water is significantly reduced. Patients have suffered burns over their entire bodies. In some cases, these burns have contributed to their deaths.

These especially tragic cases occur almost exclusively when very elderly and fragile patients, or those comatose or unconscious, are being bathed. The skin of these individuals, and of pediatric patients, is unusually sensitive. The temperature of their baths must be measured and kept below established limits. These patients should not be allowed to bathe unattended and should never be placed under running water. Regulators or valves that limit water temperature can be installed to reduce the need for constant attention to temperature.

Another source of patient burns is spills of hot food. Often, patients are unaccustomed to eating in bed and may easily spill hot coffee, tea, and soups. Nurses should be aware of patients who may be susceptible to these spills, such as children and the elderly. These patients should be supervised while they eat, and assistance may be necessary.

In addition, large facilities often utilize many electrical appliances and outlets that create the potential for electrical shock and burns. Figure 5-4 (see p. 71) summarizes safety tips to prevent injuries from these devices.

☐ Patient Smoking Guidelines

Another major cause of patient burns, and more alarmingly, of fires in the entire facility, is patient smoking. The facility must develop, implement, and enforce strict patient smoking guidelines, which every patient should know and understand. Some patient conditions—disorientation, some psychiatric problems, senility, or suicidal tendencies—may warrant severe restrictions on smoking privileges, such as allowing these patients to smoke only under close supervision.

Smoking, of course, must never be permitted in areas where oxygen is in use. Although most staff members and many patients are aware of this restriction, they find it difficult to approach a smoker in one of these areas and request that he or she extinguish the cigarette, especially if this person is a visitor. All staff members and patients, however, should be encouraged to speak up in these situations.

Along these lines, patients should be given the right to protest being placed in the same room with a smoker. Sensitive situations can be handled delicately by quickly responding to the request before animosity develops. Figure 5-5 (see p. 71) shows a sample set of facility smoking regulations. (Smoking guidelines and fire safety are discussed in greater detail in chapter 7.)

□ Medication Errors

Among the other common and potentially very serious accidents in health care facilities are medication errors. These, too, can be avoided primarily through commonsense measures and slow, deliberate pacing. To minimize medication errors, the responsibilities of all those involved in the prescribing, filling, and administering of medication should be adequately defined. This includes the attending physician and the pharmacist, as well as the attending nurse.

The attending physician must issue written medication orders. In the case of verbal orders, the physician is responsible for countersigning them within 48 hours. All orders must be legible, clear, and concise and include the patient's full name, the dosage, the time and duration of the prescription, and the name of the drug. The physician is responsible for ensuring that others fully understand his or her orders and must clarify any ambiguity.

The pharmacist bears the responsibility of preparing and dispensing all medications exactly according to the prescribing physician's orders. The pharmacist should always contact the physician when orders are unclear, and should never guess. The pharmacist must keep accurate records of the supplies of drugs and report any irregularities.

The attending nurse has the responsibility to administer medications, except when the physician is legally the only one allowed to administer the drug. To prevent medication errors at this stage, the nurse should first realize that accurate drug administration requires a careful procedure that must be done slowly and deliberately. Rushing is a frequent contributor to medication errors. Part of this cautious process includes checking all prescriptions in the order book to ensure that there are orders for the medication and that these orders have not changed.

Nurses should also keep all medications in their original containers and ensure that the labels remain intact. Labels must include the prescription number; the name, strength, and quantity of the drug; the patient's, the physician's, and the pharmacist's names; directions for use; appropriate cautionary labels; and the date of issue. Labels missing any of this information should be returned to the pharmacy.

Nurses should follow a step-by-step process for administering medication that includes at least the following steps:

1. Wash your hands before preparing medicines.
2. Correctly identify all medications under good light before measuring

them. Read the label three times:
- When removing the container from the locked cabinet
- Before measuring
- When replacing the container in the storage cabinet

3. Correctly measure all medications when they are not dispensed by unit doses in the pharmacy (although the unit dose system is recommended by the Joint Commission).
4. Realize that some drugs, in combination, have dangerous synergistic effects. If you discover such a combination, contact the prescribing physician before administering the drug.
5. Strictly adhere to the required time schedule for the administration of all pharmaceuticals.
6. Identify patients in at least two ways before giving them the medication. First, ask their names and receive a positive response. Then double-check by looking at patients' arm bands and charts.
7. Stay with the patient until all the medicine has been consumed.

It is essential that nurses be trained in this well-thought-out procedure and that the physician and the pharmacist be aware of their equal responsibility in minimizing medication errors. All medication errors should be documented in an incident report. The safety committee should regularly review trends in medication errors, and if an increase is observed, stepped-up control measures should be implemented. This constant monitoring, in addition to the safe acts of all involved, will reduce the incidence of these very risky occurrences.

☐ Special Considerations for Elderly Patients

The fastest-growing age group in America today consists of individuals over age 65. In what has been called the "graying of America," people are living longer than ever before, and in larger numbers. This trend can only be expected to continue as the baby boom generation reaches middle age and old age. It has a great bearing on health care. Older people experience a considerably greater number of health problems than their younger counterparts. Trends indicate that the United States will require 500,000 more long-term care beds by the end of this century (National Safety Council, *Long Term Care Safety Management Manual: A Handbook for Practical Application.* Chicago: National Safety Council, p. VII.). Acute care facilities will feel the effects of these demographics, too, as more elderly people come in for short-term treatment.

Many of these patients will be in surprisingly good mental and physical condition. However, the greater number of senior citizens increases the likelihood that facilities will encounter more patients who are senile, physically disabled, and often depressed. Because of this, all types of health care facilities should plan to attend to the special needs of the elderly. In elderly patients, vision often is not good; anxiety and isolation may cause disorientation or, sometimes, senility; their balance may be delicate; they may have poor circulation, making them prone to dizziness; some are incontinent, which presents safety issues as well as considerations of maintaining the patient's dignity; and many take drugs that may make them more susceptible to a variety of accidents.

Because of these special problems, many facilities have found that educating the staff about the elderly promotes understanding and compassion. The facility can have someone knowledgeable about aging discuss its effects and ways personnel can alleviate problems. For example, in many cases, shadows will confuse an elderly person, causing him or her to misjudge a step and fall. Many confused elderly patients wander and leave the facility without anyone noticing. Patients have died of exposure or from being hit by a car while wandering. In addition, abuse and neglect are more common with elderly patients, whose unresponsiveness or disabilities may frustrate staff members. A good staff education program can prevent these harmful and costly incidents.

Beyond general education, nursing home staff and hospital personnel who care for the elderly should be specifically trained in geriatric care. Treatment and care of the elderly can differ greatly from acute care for younger patients. Besides safety and liability prevention, staff trained in geriatrics will be equipped to deal with the deep emotional concerns and unique health conditions of older patients. This training will appreciably affect the quality of care the facility offers to this burgeoning sector of the population.

Patient safety should be at the heart of the safety program. The patient has come to the facility with the hopes not only of being healed but of staying in a safe environment and of being treated kindly and with respect. In setting out to deliver health care, the facility has made a commitment to serve its community through high-quality patient care. Without basic protection from accidents, patient care is at best marred and at worst negated.

☐ Conclusion

The facility must preserve the safety of patients through protection from accidents that result from improper use of restraints, unsuccessful lifting techniques, slips, falls, burns, and medication errors. Instead of just following checklists for basic safety, the facility must incorporate a philosophy that emphasizes the importance of safety and compassion in patient treatment. Only through integrating these elements into a system of total care can the facility fulfill its obligation to serve the community.

Figure 5-1. Patient Evaluation Form

We are listening.

Please tell us about your hospital stay. We would like to know how it was—so that we can continue to improve our service for future patients. Expertise in medicine is crucial, but it is important also that the physician's efforts are complemented with good care by the hospital staff. You know from experience the difference it can make.

_____ Hospital has always taken pride in giving more than technically good patient care. We want warm and considerate care—the kind that helps any patient to feel better faster. We want honest opinions on the care you received here, so we have formulated this questionnaire. We are asking you to fill it out as soon as you feel up to it.

Feel free to identify yourself or not. For your convenience, we have enclosed a self-addressed prepaid envelope.

For the medical staff, employees, and volunteers of _____ Hospital, and for the patients who will benefit in the future—thank you for your cooperation.

How are we doing? Please rate the following:	Excellent	Good	Fair	Poor
Food				
Nursing care				
Courtesy				
Answers to your questions				
General care				
Comfort and temperature of your room				
Admissions staff				
Emergency room staff (if admitted there)				
Visiting hours and rules				
Other (specify)				

Is there a complaint or problem you want us to know about?
Briefly, what is the difficulty?

_____

_____

_____

Would you like someone from the Executive Office to look into this and report back to you?
Yes _____ No _____

Name _____

Location_____ Date Admitted_____

Source: Reprinted, with permission, from Bader & Associates, Inc. *Patient Safety Manual.* Chicago: American College of Surgeons, 1979, p. 69.

Figure 5-2. A Four-Step Approach to Restraint

1. Evaluate

- What characteristics is the patient displaying? Violent behavior? Falls from the bed or wheelchair? Self-destructiveness?
- Has the patient acted this way in the past?
- Does the patient's current behavior match predetermined criteria for restraint?
- Are there indications that the patient may resist restraint?
- Might it be possible to defuse the situation so that restraint is unnecessary?

2. Plan

- How quickly must the patient be restrained?
- How and with what is the patient to be restrained?
- Do we have the staff and equipment assembled before implementation?
- Do all the team members know the plan of action?

3. Implement

- Explain to the patient what will be done.
- Work together as a team.
- Minimize the audience. If possible, move the patient to a less public area before restraining.
- Treat the patient with dignity and respect.
- After restraining the patient, explain to him or her the reasons for the restraints and when they will be removed. Check the restraints and the patient frequently.

4. Document

- Detail in an incident report what occurred, what restraining measures were used, and the authorization received.
- Chart the incident, including the times the restrained patient was checked.
- Regularly review restraining incidents and learn from mistakes.

Figure 5-3. Daily Patient Fall-Prevention List

Date: ____________________ Unit: ____________________

Date Listed	Time Listed	Name	Age	Room No.	Reason Listed	R.N. Initials

Comments: ____________________

____

[The following is] to be completed by Head Nurse or designated R.N. at end of 24-hour period.

Total Number of Patient Falls	Number of Falls by Patients Listed	Number of Falls by Patients Not Listed	Number of Incident Reports	Signature of Head Nurse or Designated R.N.

Source: Reprinted, with permission, from Wade, R. D. *Risk Management—HPL, Hospital Professional Liability Primer.* Columbus, OH: Ohio Hospital Insurance Co., 1983.

Figure 5-4. Electrical Appliance Safety Measures

Heating pads and hot-water bottles

- Never place a heating pad or hot-water bottle directly against an unconscious person, a person in shock, an infant, or a dressing.
- Check the temperature of pads and bottles. Temperatures should never exceed 130° F (54.4° C) for adults and 120° F (48.8° C) for children.
- Check skin temperature shortly after applying a pad or bottle. Do not accept the patient's opinion on his or her comfort.
- Check soundness of each item before use. Heating pads are electrical appliances and subject to all regulations set for electrical equipment.
- Use tape, binders, or straps to keep units in place. Do not use pins or clamps.
- Use heating pad only on low setting.

Infrared lamps and light cradles

- Use infrared lamps and light cradles only on the physician's orders.
- If the site to be treated is near the head, protect the patient's eyes with a towel or washcloth.
- Place the equipment at least 18 inches from the patient's body. In a light cradle only a 25-watt bulb is used.
- Ensure that equipment has guards.
- Attend the patient the entire time the equipment is in use. The attendant must be a staff member, not a visitor.
- Inspect wiring and connections daily.

Steam inhalators

- Inspect the steam inhalator equipment before using it to be sure it is filled with water.
- Prevent hot vapor from concentrating on the patient's body.
- Make sure the equipment does not overheat.
- Do not place steam inhalators on bedside tables where patients may accidentally knock them over.

All burns require immediate attention and notification of the patient's physician.

Personal electrical appliances

- Use of personal electrical appliances should be limited.
- Elderly persons, children, and patients with psychiatric conditions should be closely supervised while using personal electrical appliances.
- Check these appliances when they are brought in and, for long-term care residents, regularly thereafter for worn wiring, connections, and plugs.

Figure 5-5. Facility Smoking Regulations

The hospital restricts and discourages the smoking of cigarettes, pipes, and cigars by employees, volunteers, visitors, and patients. Smoking is restricted for patients under psychiatric care, alcoholism treatment, or treatment for drug overdose or ingestion. Smoking is forbidden in the following locations and under the following circumstances:

- In all areas of the hospital where flammable gases such as oxygen are in use or are stored
- In all areas where combustible supplies or materials are stored
- In elevators
- In surgical and obstetrical suites, with the exception of specific dressing rooms and lounges
- In any area where employees are in direct contact with patients
- By any patient on antidepressant or sleep-inducing medication

In addition to these regulations, the following smoking regulations are in effect:

- In the assignment of rooms, all efforts will be made to separate those who smoke from those who do not.
- Ambulatory patients should not smoke in bed.
- Signs posted throughout the premises mark areas where smoking is forbidden or permitted.
- Smoking by patients is to be supervised by appropriate patient care personnel.
- The sale of smoking materials on hospital premises is discouraged.

Chapter 6

Hazardous and Infectious Materials Management

Along with rapid advances in treatment and laboratory methods have come serious new threats to the safety of the health care facility's environment. Drugs and other substances with beneficial effects may also possess the ability to harm human health and the environment. At the same time, the problem of patient waste is being viewed in a new light as regulations tighten and society's attitude changes. Even building materials may contain dangerous substances; the very structure of the facility may bear inherent risks for inhabitants. Partially because of this wide variety of risks from hazardous (chemical) materials, the National Institute for Occupational Safety and Health has recognized health care facilities as one of the more dangerous places to work.

Facilities need a comprehensive program, one that embodies an integrated approach to hazardous and infectious materials and wastes. Depending on the facility, this program may be the responsibility of an individual specifically chosen for this task, or it may be incorporated in the safety program. Whatever its structure, the program should coordinate a response to all dangerous substances used in the facility, rather than approaching them in a piecemeal fashion. Table 6-1 (see p. 90) lists some hazardous materials and where they can be found within the institution. Through coordination, the risks from hazardous and infectious materials can be significantly reduced.

□ Joint Commission Requirements

The Joint Commission on Accreditation of Healthcare Organizations (Joint Commission) publishes a number of specific requirements for the health care facility's hazardous materials program. It places great emphasis on the existence of policies and procedures that relate to all aspects of hazardous and infectious materials management. These policies and procedures must be reviewed and updated at least annually by different committees, according to the type of hazard. Policies and procedures that govern the following hazardous substances are reviewed by the respective committees:

- Chemical and physical hazards are reviewed by the safety committee.
- Infectious materials are reviewed by the infection control committee.
- Radioactive substances are reviewed by the radiation safety committee.

All personnel required to handle hazardous materials and wastes must receive training specific to the materials they encounter. In addition, the facility's hazardous materials program must address not only hazardous materials in solid and liquid form but also dangerous gases. Hazardous gas precautions must include control of waste gas levels in areas such as surgical suites and in departments such as central supply and pathology.

Similarly, the program must prevent the contamination of patient care areas, food preparation areas, and serving areas by waste-compaction and storage areas. Finally, the Joint Commission requires compliance with all federal, state, and local hazardous/infectious materials standards.

□ Hazard Communication Standard

A comprehensive hazardous materials management plan begins before the chemicals arrive at the facility. It requires that staff members record what chemicals are being used in which department, their hazards, and other pertinent information. It mandates that employees be trained in the proper ways to handle the harmful materials in order to reduce risks to their safety and health.

In the mid-1970s, the Occupational Safety and Health Administration (OSHA) noticed that growing numbers of employees were working with hazardous chemicals unknowingly. In many cases, even the employers knew little or nothing about the chemicals used in the plant. Employees could not protect themselves from the hazards of these substances because they knew so little about them. Alarmed at this situation, OSHA began work on a rule that would wipe out this ignorance and its potentially lethal effects.

In November 1983, after years of research and planning, OSHA published the Hazard Communication Standard. The standard proposed that a worker has a "right to know" (a term that soon identified the standard) what chemicals he or she handles or works around.

The overall goal of the rule was to reduce the incidence of chemical-related illnesses and injuries in the manufacturing industries. It soon became evident, however, that even nonmanufacturing organizations and businesses such as health care facilities, schools, and retailers use hazardous chemicals that may jeopardize the health of employees. In August 1987, OSHA expanded coverage of the Hazard Communication Standard to all industries, including health care facilities.

In ensuring workers' "right to know," the standard requires several specific actions of employers. The major requirements are these:

1. *Hazard determination.* This is the one part of the Hazard Communication Standard that still pertains primarily to manufacturers and importers of hazardous chemicals. *Hazard determination* refers to extensive research these businesses must conduct on the hazards of the chemicals they manufacture or sell. Businesses must regularly review and update this research to maintain accuracy. The results of the hazard determination are then used to write Material Safety Data Sheets for each chemical.
2. *Material Safety Data Sheets (MSDSs).* Material Safety Data Sheets are documents that provide detailed information on chemicals, including their hazards, personal protective equipment to be used, and emergency

procedures to be followed. Manufacturers and importers must print these (based on their hazard determinations) and send them to employers. The Occupational Safety and Health Administration requires the employer to make the MSDSs available to all employees in the relevant work areas. Workers must also be trained in reading and using them. Material Safety Data Sheets comprise a crucial component of the employee's right to know. They should be a ready source of information for employees to use in becoming informed and in protecting themselves. Figure 6-1 (see p. 84) shows a sample MSDS form.

3. *Container labeling.* Employees must ensure that all chemicals in the facility are labeled with the identity of the chemicals and proper health warnings. Most chemicals come to the facility labeled, but some labels may not include all the necessary information. Moreover, chemicals are often repoured into containers not labeled for that chemical. Health care facilities should initiate a procedure for ensuring that all chemicals are properly labeled.
4. *Hazardous chemical list.* Facilities must compile a list of all the chemicals they use or produce and make this available to employees.
5. *Employee information and training.* Under the Hazard Communication Standard, employers must provide extensive information and training. Employees must be trained in:
   - What the standard requires
   - What chemicals they may be exposed to in their work
   - Where the MSDSs, lists of chemicals, and a description of the written hazard communication program are located
   - The hazards of the chemicals in their areas
   - How to recognize and handle the chemicals in their areas
   - The use of protective measures
   - The use of the facility's written hazard communication program
6. *Written hazard communication program.* The facility must explain in writing how it proposes to comply with these regulations. The resulting document is called the written hazard communication program and acts as the handbook for the facility's program of compliance.

The Occupational Safety and Health Administration can exact penalties and fines for failure to comply with the right-to-know standard. Along with the protection from regulatory censure, implementing a hazard communication program also provides a strong foundation for hazardous waste management and other precautions. The MSDSs and hazardous chemical list allow for easier tracking of chemicals when they become wastes, and employees should already be trained in where to go for information and how to protect themselves. Compliance with the Hazard Communication Standard will assist in Joint Commission accreditation, as it places more and more emphasis on limiting the hazards from dangerous substances.

☐ Hazardous Waste

After their use, hazardous chemicals become hazardous waste. Although they are wastes, the materials still pose risks to the facility and environment. They must be contained appropriately and stored under the proper conditions. Most important, facilities cannot dispose of these wastes in a haphazard manner. Improper disposal can pollute the environment and endanger the life and health of people and wildlife.

As discussed in chapter 2, the Environmental Protection Agency (EPA) has the power under several laws to prevent such damage to the environment. The law of primary interest to health care facilities is the Resource Conservation and Recovery Act (RCRA). Health care facilities must realize that they generate hazardous waste in quantities significant enough to be covered by RCRA. Xylene, azides, formaldehyde, and mercury represent just a few of the waste chemicals health care facilities produce in everyday operation.

Definition

According to RCRA, a discarded material is a hazardous waste if:

1. It appears on one or more hazardous substance *lists* published by the EPA.
2. It has any of the following *characteristics:*
   - *Ignitability.* The waste is easily combustible or flammable (for example, benzene, xylene, ethyl ether, acetone).
   - *Corrosivity.* The waste dissolves metals or other materials or burns the skin (for example, hydrochloric acid, sodium hydroxide, sulfuric acid).
   - *Reactivity.* The waste is "explosive," or unstable, or undergoes rapid or violent chemical reaction with water or other materials [for example, hydrogen peroxide (30%), picric acid, azides, perchloric acid (60%)].
   - *Toxicity.* The waste may release toxic substances into groundwater or engender a hazard to human health or the environment (for example, compounds containing lead, mercury, chromium, silver, or arsenic).
3. It is an *acutely hazardous* waste as defined by the EPA (for example, cyanide and cyanide compounds, arsenate and arsenic compounds, sodium azide, parathion, osmium tetroxide).

Generator Status

Every facility must conduct a survey to determine the quantity and type of hazardous waste it uses. From this, the facility determines its "generator status." Four generator classes are recognized by the EPA: (1) up to 100 kg of nonacutely hazardous waste per month, (2) between 100 kg (220 lbs) and 1,000 kg (2,200 lbs) of nonacutely hazardous waste per month, (3) greater than 1,000 kg of nonacutely hazardous waste per month, and (4) greater than 1 kg (2.2 lbs) of acutely hazardous waste per month. Most health care facilities fall under the "small-quantity generator" category, generating from 100 to 1,000 kg (2,200 lbs) of nonacutely hazardous waste per month. Each facility must determine its own category and understand the regulations that apply.

If the facility generates more than 100 kg of hazardous waste per month, it must obtain an EPA Identification Number. To acquire this number, contact your state hazardous waste management agency or EPA regional office and ask for Form 8700-12 (see figure 6-2 on p. 86 for a sample form). When the EPA receives the filled-out form, it will assign the facility an EPA Identification Number.

Storage

Containers used to store hazardous waste should only be large enough to hold amounts for short periods. Nonbreakable containers are preferred. Once they have been contained, the wastes may not be stored without a permit unless they are kept under 180 days for small-quantity generators that ship their wastes less than 200 miles for disposal or 270 days for small-quantity generators that ship their wastes farther away.

In addition, while in storage, containers should be protected through inspections, security, appropriate room temperature, and accurate labeling. Attention should be paid to the types of wastes stored together or in close proximity. Some wastes are incompatible and may create potentially violent reactions when stored improperly.

Disposal

The facility must have policies and procedures for preparing its waste for disposal. Once these are established, the best method(s) of disposal must be determined. There are many alternatives, such as on-site treatment and disposal, reclamation, neutralization, and recycling. Table 6-2 (see p. 91) lists some disposal options for several types of hazardous and infectious wastes, although these wastes must be treated separately.

Most facilities need to have at least some of their hazardous wastes disposed of off-site. Under RCRA, the EPA instituted a system to track wastes from the source of generation through to final disposal, from "cradle to grave." The Uniform Hazardous Waste Manifest form shown in figure 6-3 (see p. 88) is designed to accomplish this tracking. The facility that generates the waste, the transporter, and then the manager of the disposal facility must each sign and retain a copy of this document. Once the waste has been accepted by the disposal facility, the form is sent back to the facility, which must keep a copy for at least three years. However, it would be wise to retain the form indefinitely because it represents proof of the facility's compliance.

Waste Reduction

There are many specific requirements under RCRA, and complying with them may become complex, particularly for facilities with many different types and sources of waste. However, health care facilities can take positive steps to reduce the amounts of hazardous waste they produce. For example:

- Separate all nonhazardous materials from hazardous wastes at the source.
- Look into distillation, which reduces waste amounts, for such wastes as xylene and formaldehyde.
- Substitute less hazardous materials when possible. For example, a 10 percent formalin solution can be substituted for formaldehyde, a recognized carcinogen.
- Neutralize some wastes by mixing them with other substances that render the wastes inert. This must be done carefully and only by trained personnel.
- Consider lab-packing. Lab-packing is a way of carefully packaging hazardous wastes that results in a smaller number of barrels requiring disposal in a landfill. The procedure should be performed by trained personnel and a licensed disposal company.

These are just a few ways to make hazardous waste more manageable. With good planning and waste reduction techniques, hazardous waste management can become the cornerstone of the facility's hazardous materials program.

☐ SARA Title III, or "Community Right-to-Know"

As previously discussed, through application of the Hazard Communication Standard and a thorough hazardous waste management program, harmful substances can be controlled as they enter, are handled within, and leave the facility. But what happens when a hazardous substance is released into the environment, spreading illness through the community that surrounds the facility? For example, in December 1984, a Union Carbide plant in Bhopal, India, released a toxic gas into the environment, killing over 2,000 people and permanently disabling countless others.

Chapter 2 introduced the Superfund Amendments and Reauthorization Act (SARA). Title III of SARA sets up a system whereby local communities engage in planning to prevent such disastrous accidents and to minimize the destructive effects should such an emergency occur. The act recognizes that only through cooperation between business and the community can there be an effective and coordinated response to emergencies involving hazardous chemicals.

The primary responsibility for hospitals under Title III is in the area of emergency planning. Often referred to as "community right-to-know," Title III requires states to designate emergency planning districts, along with emergency planning committees for each district. These committees plan an organized response to be undertaken in an environmental disaster. The committees include wide-ranging representation, such as the media, community groups, health personnel, and fire protection representatives.

The planning committees begin by identifying businesses that generate certain large quantities of hazardous wastes. To help plan what will be done to treat those affected by a release of hazardous substances, hospitals near these businesses must provide representation on the local emergency planning committee. They must assist in identifying routes for transporting the sick and injured and protective measures for paramedics and other personnel. They must also develop a disaster preparedness plan for accommodating and treating large numbers of those made ill by the substance. Hospitals must be aware that they could be called to participate in this valuable community planning process.

A hazard communication program manages chemicals as they enter and are used in the facility; hazardous waste regulations manage the chemicals once they become waste; and Title III protects the community from the hazardous effects of the substances through a planned response to an environmental disaster. Treating these and the other elements of hazardous materials management as part of an integrated system will simplify and strengthen the facility's methods of control.

☐ Infectious Waste

Although managing hazardous chemicals and wastes is crucial, infectious waste management represents perhaps the greatest waste-handling challenge for most health care facilities. This is particularly true due to recent shifts in societal conditions, attitudes, and regulations.

Perhaps foremost among these changes is the emergence of AIDS as a major health issue. As the number of people infected and sick with the disease continues to escalate, health care facilities of all types will have to treat AIDS patients. The lethal nature of the disease has sparked fear, often irrational, in health care workers and in the general public. Also, medical waste (including vials of AIDS-tainted blood) has recently washed up on beaches along the northeastern U.S. coast. Fear of AIDS, compounded by discovery of medical wastes on beaches, set off a public outcry. Legislators have responded to this pressure by calling for stricter infectious waste procedures. In reaction, regulatory agencies have issued more stringent requirements for health care facilities.

Among these new requirements is the Centers for Disease Control's (CDC's) "universal precautions." As mentioned in chapter 4, universal precautions refers to the assumption that all body fluids or tissues are potentially infectious. This CDC recommendation has been interpreted to mean that most, if not all, patient-contact wastes should be treated as infectious. If this were translated into actual practice, officials estimate that the percentage of facility waste considered infectious would rise to 70 to 90 percent. However, the CDC has recently explained that universal precautions should not be taken as a requirement that all patient waste be treated as infectious. Although the effect of the CDC's recommendations on waste remains a matter of some debate, it is clear that universal precautions will at least prompt facilities to be more cautious in their infectious waste management procedures.

Regulatory movement in the infectious waste area continues at a rapid pace. Whereas the major source of regulation is currently state agencies, new legislation may result in federal requirements in the near future. Health care facilities should prepare themselves for stricter standards by expanding their infectious waste management programs now. Each facility should check with the state agency that regulates infectious waste to find out the current status of state and local requirements.

Despite changes and differences in state regulations, some infectious waste guidelines are recommended for all health care facilities:

- Obtain CDC and EPA infectious waste guidelines (see chapter 2 for information on how to contact these agencies).
- Classify infectious waste by using the categories recommended by the EPA (see table 6-3 on p. 92).
- Separate infectious waste from other waste.
- Contain infectious waste in plastic bags or other containers designated as appropriate for infectious waste and clearly marked with the universal biohazard symbol shown in figure 6-4 (see p. 89).
- Use puncture-resistant containers for sharps and bottles, and use flasks or tanks for liquids.
- Minimize storage time and clearly mark storage areas.
- Avoid containers susceptible to tearing or breaking.
- Establish standard operating procedures for treatment of infectious waste.
- Monitor treatment of infectious waste.
- Obtain any necessary licenses for on-site treatment, such as incinerator permits.
- Contact state and local governments for disposal options.
- Develop a plan for response to infectious waste emergencies, including:
  - Spill cleanup
  - Personal protective measures
  - Alternative arrangements for waste storage and treatment during equipment failure (such as incinerator breakdown)
- Require those handling infectious waste to use proper personal protective equipment, such as surgical latex gloves.

Commonsense measures, along with a progressive attitude of anticipation, will protect the facility today and prepare it for tomorrow.

☐ Cytotoxic Drugs

Cytotoxic drugs, also called antineoplastic agents and chemotherapy drugs, are used in the chemotherapeutic treatment of cancer. Figure 6-5 (see p. 89) lists some commonly used cytotoxic drugs. Cytotoxic drugs are designed to limit or reverse the growth of malignant tumors. To do this, many cytotoxic drugs must create change at the most basic level of cellular activity. The powerful potential of these drugs can make them very hazardous to those not being treated for cancer. In healthy individuals, in fact, antineoplastic agents have been linked with cancer, organ damage, sterility, and birth defects. In addition, acute effects include irritation of the skin and mucous membranes, especially the eyes, and tissue necrosis (the "death" of tissue).

Guidance for and regulation of the handling of cytotoxic drugs come from several sources. Many cytotoxic drugs appear on EPA hazardous substances lists. The Occupational Safety and Health Administration has issued guidelines for the use of chemotherapeutic drugs. Moreover, OSHA's General Duty clause (explained in chapter 2) requires employers to provide a safe and healthful workplace for employees. Harmful exposure to antineoplastic drugs could constitute a violation of this clause.

Health care employees who could potentially be exposed to chemotherapy drugs are many, including physicians and employees from:

- Pharmacy
- Nursing
- Housekeeping
- Laundry
- Oncology
- Pathology
- Emergency room
- Morgue

Training should be in place for all affected staff on safe methods of handling antineoplastic drugs. In addition, detailed policies and procedures should be written for all tasks that pose the potential for cytotoxic exposure, including mixing the drugs, administering them, handling specimens from patients undergoing chemotherapy, disposing of chemotherapy drugs and contaminated waste, cleaning areas where patients receive chemotherapy, cleaning spills of cytotoxic drugs, and disposing of contaminated wastes. Although all of these procedures cannot be discussed within the scope of this book, some guidelines for working with or around antineoplastic drugs are given below:

- Refer to OSHA Instruction PUB 8-1.1, "Work Practice Guidelines for Personnel Dealing with Cytotoxic (Antineoplastic) Drugs" and the National Study Commission on Cytotoxic Exposure (NSCCE) guidelines for handling antineoplastic drugs.
- Label all cytotoxic drugs and wastes and segregate this waste from infectious waste. A yellow background with black lettering is becoming accepted as signifying cytotoxic waste. It helps distinguish antineoplastic drugs from "red-bagged" infectious waste.
- Syringes and needles should never be cut, and all sharps should be disposed of using a puncture-resistant container.
- The facility may wish not to allow pregnant or breast-feeding women to handle cytotoxic drugs at all.
- Urine and excrement from patients undergoing chemotherapy should be

handled only when using proper personal protective equipment.
- Those handling cytotoxic drugs or wastes contaminated by cytotoxic drugs, including laundry and housekeeping personnel, should be required to wear surgical latex gloves and approved protective disposable gowns.
- Employees should always wash their hands after handling cytotoxic drugs or cytotoxic-contaminated items, even if gloves were worn.
- Those mixing chemotherapy drugs should be provided with a Class II, Type A or B biological safety cabinet.
- Smoking, drinking, applying cosmetics, and eating in areas where these drugs are prepared, stored, or used should be strictly prohibited. The employee can ingest harmful amounts of the drug through any of these activities.
- Spills and breakages should be cleaned up immediately by a properly protected person trained in the appropriate procedures. Access to spill areas must be restricted.
- Most chemical inactivators may produce hazardous by-products and should not be applied to the spilled material.
- All contaminated surfaces should be thoroughly cleaned with detergent solution and then wiped clean with water.

Cytotoxic drugs can have serious effects on exposed individuals, including long-term consequences that may not appear for years, even decades. Consequently, a strong possibility for liability exists. To avoid the potentially tragic conditions linked with exposure and to reduce the facility's vulnerability to litigation, a thorough program of control must be in place. This program will contribute significantly to the maintenance of a safe and healthful work environment.

☐ Reproductive Health Hazards

In addition to cytotoxic drugs, other substances used in the operation of a health care facility can have negative effects on reproduction. These effects include birth defects, infertility, impotence, spontaneous abortion (miscarriage), and increased infant mortality. Reproductive health hazards can affect both men and women, so both sexes should be protected.

As research into the hazards of chemicals progresses, some long-used substances are being linked with harmful effects on the reproductive system. These effects may require years, even generations, to appear. As information becomes available, health care facilities should identify the reproductive toxins to which their employees may be exposed. Substances commonly used in health care facilities that can cause damage to the reproductive system include ethylene oxide (EtO), fluorinated hydrocarbons, cytotoxic drugs, mercury, nitrous oxide, formaldehyde, and various ingredients in cleaning solutions. Also polychlorinated biphenyls (PCBs), which may be present in the transformers of some older facilities, have also been linked with reproductive damage. Finally, although it is not a chemical, the X-ray process poses reproductive risks to pregnant women.

A survey should be conducted to determine what reproductive toxins are being used where. Jobs that entail handling of these substances should also be identified. The facility must write and implement strict policies and procedures for each task that requires handling of the materials. These policies and procedures should include:

- Possibly, a requirement that female personnel in affected areas and jobs report as soon as possible suspected or confirmed pregnancy, or the intention to become pregnant. This information must be used only to protect the employee. Restrictions on employment or the responsibilities of any personnel should be avoided. Instead, attention should be paid to ways of protecting employees without placing unnecessary restrictions on them.

- A policy that pregnant employees will either not be allowed to handle or work around the substance(s) or will be adequately protected when handling or working around them.
- Information and training on the hazards and protective measures for these materials.
- Equal attention to men and women.
- Attention to housekeeping and laundry personnel and others who may also be exposed during cleanup or other work.
- Medical surveillance for all employees accidentally exposed to these substances or exposed through routine job tasks.

In the attempt to protect workers, employers should avoid sex discrimination either in hiring or in the work employees are allowed to do. Although the facility may be trying to protect its workers, unwarranted restrictions on certain employees may be construed as discriminatory. The facility must find a middle road between protection and failure to provide equal access. With some careful planning, such a path can and must be discovered because, as with cytotoxic drugs, it is imperative that health care facilities address the reproductive health hazards posed to their employees.

☐ Asbestos: Health Effects and Management Considerations

Asbestos is a fibrous material with a multitude of uses, most notably insulation and fireproofing. Certain of its traits, such as strength and heat resistance, make asbestos a very versatile material. Because of this versatility and its effectiveness in various uses, consumption of the material in this century has steadily increased with time. By 1975, the United States was using 800,000 tons of asbestos a year. Consequently, a majority of buildings built during the early 1970s contain some kind of asbestos. Table 6-4 (see p. 92) is a summary of asbestos-containing products.

As asbestos use became prevalent, however, scientists began to uncover a link between certain diseases and asbestos exposure. With further study, this link grew stronger, and by the mid-1970s, the EPA had banned many asbestos-containing products. Today, most asbestos-containing materials are either severely restricted or outlawed.

The major diseases associated with asbestos exposure are:

1. *Asbestosis.* Asbestosis occurs when the tiny fibers present in asbestos-containing material are inhaled. The disease is characterized by scarring of the lung from these fibers and a reduction of lung capacity. Asbestosis is severely disabling and can be fatal.
2. *Lung cancer.* Employees exposed to industrial concentrations of asbestos have a risk of contracting lung cancer five times greater than those not exposed to asbestos. Those who smoke and work with asbestos in high concentrations are 50 times more likely to develop the disease.
3. *Mesothelioma.* Mesothelioma is a cancer of the mesothelia, the chest

cavity lining. Most cases have been traced directly to a history of asbestos exposure. The disease is always fatal.

Although these diseases are most often found in those who worked consistently with asbestos, no known safe level of exposure exists. This is important because, although most asbestos-containing products are now banned, many buildings built in the 1960s and 1970s still contain the dangerous material. When the asbestos in these products, such as roof and floor tiles, is disturbed and released, it can be carried through vents and dispersed throughout the building.

Employees who worked in buildings documented to contain asbestos and who later developed asbestos-linked diseases have sued building owners and employers. Although the limits of responsibility are still being tested in the courts and legislatures, this may represent a serious vulnerability as well as a health hazard. It seems likely that legislation will be passed to require owners of all buildings either to remove or somehow contain the hazard. Managers and those with safety responsibilities must inform their superiors of these risks and ensure that measures are taken to abate the hazards. Sound preparation will make the transition to an asbestos-free environment smoother when the time comes.

□ Conclusion

This chapter could only hint at the multitude of risks engendered by the use of hazardous materials in health care facilities. Taken together, hazardous and infectious materials and wastes constitute perhaps the single greatest threat to the health of employees and the safety and financial stability of the facility. For this reason, health care facilities, including nursing homes, must respond to present risks and anticipate new ones. The institution and those within it, as well as the surrounding environment, can be protected through an integrated hazardous and infectious materials management program.

Figure 6-1. Material Safety Data Sheet

Material Safety Data Sheet

May be used to comply with OSHA's Hazard Communication Standard, 29CFR 1910. 1200. Standard must be consulted for specific requirements.

QUICK IDENTIFIER
Common Name: (used on label and list)

SECTION 1 -

Manufacturer's Name

Address	Emergency Telephone No.
City, State, and ZIP	Other Information Calls
Signature of Person Responsible for Preparation (Optional)	Date Prepared

SECTION 2 – HAZARDOUS INGREDIENTS/IDENTITY

Hazardous Component(s) (chemical & common name(s))	OSHA PEL	ACGIH TLV	Other Exposure Limits	% (optional)	CAS NO.

SECTION 3 - PHYSICAL & CHEMICAL CHARACTERISTICS

Boiling Point	Specific Gravity (H_2O=1)	Vapor Pressure (mm Hg)
Vapor Density (Air = 1)		
Solubility in Water	Reactivity in Water	
Appearance and Odor	Melting Point	

SECTION 4 – FIRE & EXPLOSION DATA

Flash Point F. C.	Method Used	Flammable Limits in Air % by Volume	LEL Lower	UEL Upper
Auto-Ignition Temperature	Extinguisher Media			

Special Fire Fighting Procedures

Unusual Fire and Explosion Hazards

Note: This is page 1 of a two-page form.

Figure 6-1. (Continued)

SECTION 5 – PHYSICAL HAZARDS (REACTIVITY DATA)

Stability Unstable ☐ Conditions
Stable ☐ to Avoid

Incompatability
(Materials to Avoid)

Hazardous
Decomposition Products

Hazardous Polymerization May Occur ☐ Will Not Occur ☐ Conditions to Avoid

SECTION 6 – HEALTH HAZARDS

1. Acute 2. Chronic

Signs and
Symptoms of Exposure

Medical Conditions Generally
Aggravated by Exposure

Chemical Listed as Carcinogen or Potential Carcinogen | National Toxicology Program Yes ☐ No ☐ | I.A.R.C. Monographs Yes ☐ No ☐ | OSHA Yes ☐ No ☐

Emergency and
First Aid Procedures

ROUTES OF ENTRY
1. Inhalation
2. Eyes
3. Skin
4. Ingestion

SECTION 7 - SPECIAL PRECAUTIONS AND SPILL/LEAK PROCEDURES

Precautions to be Taken
in Handling and Storage

Other
Precautions

Steps to be Taken in Case
Material is Released or Spilled

Waste Disposal
Methods (Consult federal, state, and local regulations)

SECTION 8 – SPECIAL PROTECTION INFORMATION/CONTROL MEASURES

Respiratory Protection
(Specify Type)

Ventilation | Local Exhaust | Mechanical (General) | Special | Other

Protective Gloves | Eye Protection

Other Protective
Clothing or Equipment

Work/Hygienic Practices

IMPORTANT
Do not leave any blank spaces. If required information is unavailable, unknown, or does not apply, so indicate.

CU-F1R Printed by Labelmaster, Division of American Labelmark Company, Inc. Chicago, IL 60646-6719 1-800-621-5808 • (321) 478-0900

Source: Reprinted, with permission, from Labelmaster Division, American Labelmark Co., Chicago.

Figure 6-2. EPA Notification of Hazardous Waste Activity Form

Please print or type with ELITE type *(12 characters per inch)* in the unshaded areas only

Form Approved. OMB No. 2050-0028. Expires 9-30-88.
GSA No. 0246-EPA-OT

United States Environmental Protection Agency
Washington, DC 20460

EPA Notification of Hazardous Waste Activity

Please refer to the *Instructions for Filing Notification* before completing this form. The information requested here is required by law *(Section 3010 of the Resource Conservation and Recovery Act).*

For Official Use Only

Comments

C C

Installation's EPA ID Number | Approved | Date Received *(yr. mo. day)*

C F | T/A C 1

I. Name of Installation

II. Installation Mailing Address

Street or P.O. Box

C 3

City or Town | State | ZIP Code

C 4

III. Location of Installation

Street or Route Number

C 5

City or Town | State | ZIP Code

C 6

IV. Installation Contact

Name and Title *(last, first, and job title)* | Phone Number *(area code and number)*

C 2

V. Ownership

A. Name of Installation's Legal Owner | B. Type of Ownership *(enter code)*

C R

VI. Type of Regulated Waste Activity *(Mark 'X' in the appropriate boxes. Refer to instructions.)*

A. Hazardous Waste Activity

- ☐ 1a. Generator ☐ 1b. Less than 1,000 kg/mo.
- ☐ 2. Transporter
- ☐ 3. Treater/Storer/Disposer
- ☐ 4. Underground Injection
- ☐ 5. Market or Burn Hazardous Waste Fuel *(enter 'X' and mark appropriate boxes below)*
  - ☐ a. Generator Marketing to Burner
  - ☐ b. Other Marketer
  - ☐ c. Burner

B. Used Oil Fuel Activities

- ☐ 6. Off-Specification Used Oil Fuel *(enter 'X' and mark appropriate boxes below)*
  - ☐ a. Generator Marketing to Burner
  - ☐ b. Other Marketer
  - ☐ c. Burner
- ☐ 7. Specification Used Oil Fuel Marketer *(or On site Burner)* Who First Claims the Oil Meets the Specification

VII. Waste Fuel Burning: Type of Combustion Device *(enter 'X' in all appropriate boxes to indicate type of combustion device(s) in which hazardous waste fuel or off-specification used oil fuel is burned. See instructions for definitions of combustion devices.)*

☐ A. Utility Boiler ☐ B. Industrial Boiler ☐ C. Industrial Furnace

VIII. Mode of Transportation *(transporters only — enter 'X' in the appropriate box(es))*

☐ A. Air ☐ B. Rail ☐ C. Highway ☐ D. Water ☐ E. Other *(specify)*

IX. First or Subsequent Notification

Mark 'X' in the appropriate box to indicate whether this is your installation's first notification of hazardous waste activity or a subsequent notification. If this is not your first notification, enter your installation's EPA ID Number in the space provided below.

☐ A. First Notification ☐ B. Subsequent Notification *(complete item C)*

C. Installation's EPA ID Number

EPA Form 8700-12 (Rev. 11-85) Previous edition is obsolete. **Continue on reverse**

Note: This is page 1 of a two-page form. This form expired in September 1988. A new form was being developed but was unavailable at press time. The new form will have a different format but will bear the same number and carry essentially the same information.

Figure 6-2. (Continued)

ID — For Official Use Only

C		T/A	C
W			1

X. Description of Hazardous Wastes *(continued from front)*

A. Hazardous Wastes from Nonspecific Sources. Enter the four-digit number from 40 *CFR* Part 261.31 for each listed hazardous waste from nonspecific sources your installation handles. Use additional sheets if necessary.

1	2	3	4	5	6
7	8	9	10	11	12

B. Hazardous Wastes from Specific Sources. Enter the four-digit number from 40 *CFR* Part 261.32 for each listed hazardous waste from specific sources your installation handles. Use additional sheets if necessary.

13	14	15	16	17	18
19	20	21	22	23	24
25	26	27	28	29	30

C. Commercial Chemical Product Hazardous Wastes. Enter the four-digit number from 40 *CFR* Part 261.33 for each chemical substance your installation handles which may be a hazardous waste. Use additional sheets if necessary.

31	32	33	34	35	36
37	38	39	40	41	42
43	44	45	46	47	48

D. Listed Infectious Wastes. Enter the four-digit number from 40 *CFR* Part 261.34 for each hazardous waste from hospitals, veterinary hospitals, or medical and research laboratories your installation handles. Use additional sheets if necessary.

49	50	51	52	53	54

E. Characteristics of Nonlisted Hazardous Wastes. Mark 'X' in the boxes corresponding to the characteristics of nonlisted hazardous wastes your installation handles. *(See 40 CFR Parts 261.21 — 261.24)*

☐ 1. Ignitable *(D001)* ☐ 2. Corrosive *(D002)* ☐ 3. Reactive *(D003)* ☐ 4. Toxic *(D000)*

XI. Certification

I certify under penalty of law that I have personally examined and am familiar with the information submitted in this and all attached documents, and that based on my inquiry of those individuals immediately responsible for obtaining the information, I believe that the submitted information is true, accurate, and complete. I am aware that there are significant penalties for submitting false information, including the possibility of fine and imprisonment.

Signature	Name and Official Title *(type or print)*	Date Signed

EPA Form 8700-12 (Rev. 11-85) Reverse

Figure 6-3. Uniform Hazardous Waste Manifest Form

Please print or type. (Form designed for use on elite (12-pitch) typewriter.)

Form Approved. OMB No. 2050-0039. Expires 9-30-91

UNIFORM HAZARDOUS WASTE MANIFEST

1. Generator's US EPA ID No. | Manifest Document No. | 2. Page 1 of | Information in the shaded areas is not required by Federal law.

GENERATOR

3. Generator's Name and Mailing Address | A. State Manifest Document Number | B. State Generator's ID

4. Generator's Phone ( )

5. Transporter 1 Company Name | 6. US EPA ID Number | C. State Transporter's ID | D. Transporter's Phone

7. Transporter 2 Company Name | 8. US EPA ID Number | E. State Transporter's ID | F. Transporter's Phone

9. Designated Facility Name and Site Address | 10. US EPA ID Number | G. State Facility's ID | H. Facility's Phone

11. US DOT Description (Including Proper Shipping Name, Hazard Class and ID Number)	12. Containers		13. Total Quantity	14. Unit Wt/Vol	I. Waste No.
HM	No.	Type			
a.					
b.					
c.					
d.					

J. Additional Descriptions for Materials Listed Above | K. Handling Codes for Wastes Listed Above

15. Special Handling Instructions and Additional Information

16. **GENERATOR'S CERTIFICATION:** I hereby declare that the contents of this consignment are fully and accurately described above by proper shipping name and are classified, packed, marked, and labeled, and are in all respects in proper condition for transport by highway according to applicable international and national government regulations.

If I am a large quantity generator, I certify that I have a program in place to reduce the volume and toxicity of waste generated to the degree I have determined to be economically practicable and that I have selected the practicable method of treatment, storage, or disposal currently available to me which minimizes the present and future threat to human health and the environment; **OR**, if I am a small quantity generator, I have made a good faith effort to minimize my waste generation and select the best waste management method that is available to me and that I can afford.

Printed/Typed Name | Signature | Month Day Year

TRANSPORTER

17. Transporter 1 Acknowledgement of Receipt of Materials

Printed/Typed Name | Signature | Month Day Year

18. Transporter 2 Acknowledgement of Receipt of Materials

Printed/Typed Name | Signature | Month Day Year

FACILITY

19. Discrepancy Indication Space

20. Facility Owner or Operator: Certification of receipt of hazardous materials covered by this manifest except as noted in Item 19.

Printed/Typed Name | Signature | Month Day Year

Style F15REV-6 LABELMASTER, Div. of AMERICAN LABELMARK CO., CHICAGO, IL 60646

EPA Form 8700-22 (Rev. 9-88) Previous editions are obsolete.

Source: Reprinted, with permission, from Labelmaster Division, American Labelmark Co., Chicago, copyright Sept. 1986.

Figure 6-4. Biohazard Symbol

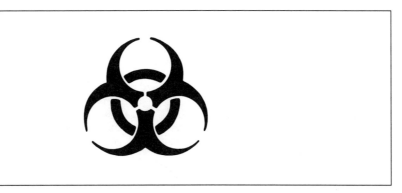

Source: Labelmaster Division, American Labelmark Co., Chicago.

Figure 6-5. Commonly Used Cytotoxic Drugs

Alkylating Agents

Cis-Platin
Cyclophosphamide
Nitrogen Mustard
Triethylene thiophosphoramide
Carmustine
Streptozocin
Busulfan
Chlorambucil
CCNU
Melphalan (Alkeran)
Myleran
Teosulfan
Uracil Mustard
Chlornaphazin
Dacarbazine

Investigationals

Azacytidine
Amsacrine
Melphalan
VM-26
Ifosfamide
Mitoxantrone
Vindesine

Antimetabolites

Cytosine Arabinoside
Fluorouracil
Methotrexate
Mercaptopurine
Azathioprime
Procarbazine

Antibiotics

Doxorubicin
Bleomycin
Dactinomycin (Actinomycin-D)
Daunorubicin
Mithramycin
Mitomycin C
Daunomycin

Mitotic Inhibitors

Vincristine
Vinblastine
Eeoposide (VP-16-213)

Miscellaneous

L-Asparaginase
Dacarbazine

Source: Reprinted, with permission, from the American Society for Hospital Engineering. *Hazardous Waste Management Strategies for Health Care Facilities.* Chicago: American Society for Hospital Engineering, 1987, p. 30.

Table 6-1. Areas of a Health Care Facility Where Hazardous Materials and Wastes May Be Found

Area	Chemical Wastes	Infectious Wastes	Sharps	Chemotherapeutic Wastes	Radioactive Wastes
Patient care area	Rare	Yes	Yes	Yes	Rare
Laboratory	Yes	Yes	Yes	Rare	Yes
Physical plant services	Yes	Rare	Yes	Rare	Rare
Laundry area	Yes	Yes	Yes	Yes	Rare
Foodservice	Yes	Rare	Yes	Rare	No
Occupational therapy/ physical therapy areas	Some	Rare	Yes	Rare	Rare
Sterile prqxaration services	Some	Some	Yes	Yes	Rare
Operating room/ intensive care units	Yes	Yes	Yes	Some	Rare
Outpatient clinic	Rare	Yes	Yes	Yes	Rare

Note: This is not an exhaustive list of all hazardous materials and wastes or of all areas where they may be found.

Source: Reprinted, with permission, from *PTSM Monograph: Managing Hazardous Wastes and Materials.* Chicago: Joint Commission on Accreditation of Healthcare Organizations, 1986, p. 17.

Table 6-2. Disposal Options for Basic Types of Waste

Types of Waste	Disposal in Sewage	Incineration	Landfill	Processing	Recycling
Chemical wastes	Sometimes appropriate.	Sometimes appropriate.	Appropriate. A special chemical landfill must be used for many chemical wastes.	Appropriate. Processing for chemical wastes is usually neutralization.	Sometimes appropriate.
Infectious wastes	Appropriate. Infectious wastes may need to be processed first.	Ideal.	Sometimes appropriate. Infectious wastes must be treated first.	Appropriate. Processing for infectious wastes is usually autoclaving.	Not appropriate.
Sharps	Not appropriate.	Sometimes appropriate.	Usually appropriate.	Sometimes appropriate. Some sharps, such as microscope slides and needles, need to be autoclaved.	Not appropriate.
Chemotherapeutic wastes	Not appropriate. Subject to state and local regulations.	Ideal.	Never appropriate.	Not appropriate.	Not appropriate.
Radioactive wastes	Sometimes appropriate.	Sometimes appropriate.	Appropriate. A special radioactive waste landfill is used for most radioactive wastes.	Appropriate. Processing for radioactive wastes is usually either compaction or letting radioactive decay take its course.	Not appropriate.

Source: Adapted, with permission, from *PTSM Monograph: Managing Hazardous Wastes and Materials.* Chicago: Joint Commission on Accreditation of Healthcare Organizations, 1986, p. 23.

Table 6-3. EPA-Designated Categories of Infectious Waste

Waste Category	Examples*
Isolation wastes	Refer to Centers for Disease Control *Guidelines for Isolation Precautions in Hospitals,* July 1983
Cultures and stocks of infectious agents and associated biologicals	Specimens from medical and pathology laboratories Cultures and stocks of infectious agents from clinical, research, and industrial laboratories; disposable culture dishes and devices used to transfer, inoculate, and mix cultures Wastes from production of biologicals Discarded live and attenuated vaccines
Human blood and blood products	Waste blood, serum, plasma, and blood products
Pathological waste	Tissues, organs, body parts, blood, and body fluids removed during surgery, autopsy, and biopsy
Contaminated sharps	Contaminated hypodermic needles, syringes, scalpel blades, pasteur pipettes, and broken glass
Contaminated animal carcasses, body parts, and bedding	Contaminated animal carcasses, body parts, and bedding of animals that were intentionally exposed to pathogens

*These materials are examples of wastes in each category. The categories are not limited to these materials.

Table 6-4. Summary of Asbestos-Containing Products

Product	Average Percent Asbestos	Binder	Dates Used
Friction products	50	Various polymers	1910–present
Plastic products			
Floor tile and sheet	20	PVC, asphalt	1950–present
Coatings and sealants	10	Asphalt	1900–present
Rigid plastics	<50	Phenolic resin	?–present
Cement pipe and sheet	20	Portland cement	1930–present
Paper products			
Roofing felt	15	Asphalt	1910–present
Gaskets	80	Various polymers	?–present
Corrugated paper pipe wrap	80	Starches, sodium silicate	1910–present
Other paper	80	Polymers, starches, silicates	1910–present
Textile products	90	Cotton, wool	1910–present
Insulating and decorative products			
Sprayed coating	50	Portland cement, silicates, organic binders	1935–1978
Troweled coating	70	Portland cement, silicates	1935–1978
Preformed pipe wrap	50	Magnesium carbonate, calcium silicate	1926–1975
Insulation board	30	Silicates	Unknown
Boiler insulation	10	Magnesium carbonate, calcium silicate	1890–1978
Other uses	<50	Many types	1900–present

Source: Reprinted from the Environmental Protection Agency, *Asbestos Waste Management Guidance,* May 1985, p. 9.

Chapter 7
Fire Safety

A well-organized system of fire safety is a vital component of the facility's safety program. Such a system embraces the two distinct, yet interrelated, elements of fire protection: prevention and response. The institution must have established and comprehensive procedures to prevent the occurrence of fire, such as good housekeeping and stringent smoking rules. It must also plan and practice how best to respond to a fire to avoid loss of life and property. In this effort, few measures are more successful than an ongoing liaison with the local fire department. Fire fighters can act as a source of information on codes and fire prevention techniques, and they may also help plan drills and in-service training. Most of all, they are the ones who would respond in a real fire emergency. For this reason alone, a productive working relationship with the local fire protection district is essential to effective fire safety.

□ Fire Safety Requirements

The National Fire Protection Association (NFPA), introduced in chapter 2, along with its two most important codes for health care—NFPA 99, *Standard for Health Care Facilities* and NFPA 101, *Life Safety Code*—is considered to be the authoritative source on fire safety. The requirements set forth by this organization are complemented by the Joint Commission on Accreditation of Healthcare Organization's (Joint Commission's) fire safety standards and the Occupational Safety and Health Administration's (OSHA's) regulations for fire protection. Together, these standards form a nexus of protection against the senseless tragedy of fire. Following are some of the most important requirements for health care facilities:

- Each patient care building must comply with the state and local codes and the appropriate edition of the *Life Safety Code.*
- A comprehensive statement of construction and fire protection must describe this compliance. However, the facility may adopt "equivalent"

measures as long as they are as effective as or better than the applicable standard.

- The facility must have a written fire plan that documents measures to prevent and respond to a fire. All fire protection measures must be documented in policies and procedures.
- Each building must have a fire alarm and fire detection system. The system should automatically activate an alarm in the event of a fire. Fire department notification must also be provided.
- Air-conditioning and heating ducts and related equipment must be installed in accordance with NFPA 90A. These systems will minimize the spread of fire and smoke in the event of fire.
- The sound of the alarm must be distinct from other paging codes and loud enough to be heard over normal operational noise levels.
- Manual fire alarm stations must be located near each required exit and at other locations so that travel distance does not exceed 200 feet.
- The electrical monitoring devices of automatic sprinkler systems must be connected to the fire alarm system. These must be tested at least annually.
- Fire extinguishers must be located so that distance to a unit never exceeds 75 feet. The fire extinguisher provided must be appropriate for the type of fire likely in that area and must be clearly identified. (Figure 7-1 on p. 102 describes fire extinguisher classifications, and table 7-1 on p. 109 lists types of extinguishers and their recommended locations.) Fire extinguishers must be inspected at least monthly and be regularly maintained, and records must be kept of inspections and maintenance.
- All fire alarm and detection systems should be tested at least quarterly.
- When buying new materials, such as bedding, draperies, furnishings, and decorations, personnel should choose items that are flame-resistant. However, staff must be advised that sending fire-resistant drapes and materials to be dry-cleaned can remove the fire-retardant finish. The facility should ensure that the launderer reapplies the finish before returning the materials.
- Wastebaskets must be constructed of noncombustible materials. Because plastic liners can increase the possibility of a fire in a noncombustible wastebasket, these should still be monitored.
- In sprinkler-protected patient care areas, the sections of privacy curtains that are within 18 inches of the ceiling must have a minimum of 1/2-inch mesh. Recent testing indicates that the sprinkler head dispersion pattern is severely hampered by curtains of fine mesh.
- Fire drills for all personnel on all shifts should be conducted at least quarterly.
- A facilitywide smoking policy should be enforced.
- Electrical safety policies must be written and enacted.
- Personnel must be regularly trained in fire safety, including response plans.
- The emergency power system must be able to provide electricity to the following systems in the event of an outage:
  - Alarm systems
  - Blood, bone, and tissue storage units
  - Obstetrical delivery rooms
  - Exit illumination
  - At least one elevator
  - Emergency care areas
  - Emergency communication systems
  - Medical air compressors
  - Medical/surgical vacuum systems
  - Newborn nurseries

— Operating rooms
— Postoperatives, recovery rooms
— Special care units

- All elevators that travel 25 feet or more above the level where fire-fighting personnel will enter must be equipped with an automatic elevator recall system. Section 7-4 of NFPA's *Life Safety Code* further explains this requirement.
- Commercial cooking equipment must be installed with proper systems to remove grease-laden vapors, in accordance with NFPA 96. Natural gas systems must have automatic shut-off valves with manual reset.
- Linen and rubbish chutes must be kept in good repair. Doors must shut and lock when released. In addition, the chutes must be provided with automatic extinguishing protection, and the chute door must have a 1 1/2-hour fire protection rating.
- The fire protection program must be reviewed and revised regularly. Solutions to problems must be determined, implemented, and documented.

These represent minimum fire safety requirements. State and local governments often promulgate their own codes, which may be stricter than OSHA, Joint Commission, or NFPA rules. Each facility should check with state and local authorities and the local fire protection district to determine what additional standards affect it.

One of the foremost lines of defense against fire does not appear in minimum standards: housekeeping. Poor housekeeping practices can contribute to the spread, and possibly even cause, of fires. Conversely, a clean and orderly facility will prevent many fires and inhibit the spread of any that do start. Carelessly discarded rags that have been in contact with a flammable liquid, such as gasoline or cleaning fluids, have been known to spark fires in health care facilities, killing many. Improperly stored hazardous materials, piles of linens left in corridors, obstructed sprinklers or fire doors, cluttered work areas, and accumulated trash can all start fires or encourage their spread. Every employee should be held accountable for keeping his or her work area clean and orderly through daily housekeeping practices. In addition, housekeeping personnel should be directed to respond promptly to spills and not allow rubbish to accumulate. (See figure 7-2 on p. 103 for a fire safety inspection checklist.)

☐ Smoking Regulations

Studies have shown that smoking is the number-one cause of fires in health care facilities (Hall, J. R. *Code Red!* Quincy, MA: National Fire Protection Association, 37:51–54, Mar. 1986.). Smoking in bed and near oxygen, carelessly disposing of cigarettes, and dropping cigarettes and matches are among the many ways smoking can set off fires. Smoking is also among the most avoidable causes of fires. A strict smoking policy that is enforced can prevent the unwarranted injury, loss of life, and property damage inflicted by smoking-related fires.

Restrictions on smoking should not only apply to patients (see chapter 5) but to staff and visitors as well. Although a complete ban on smoking may not be considered feasible or just, regulations, safety principles, and concern for the health of smokers and nonsmokers alike require that smoking be strongly discouraged. Fire training should emphasize the safety hazards posed by smoking as well as its negative health effects. The chief executive officer (CEO) or administrator should stress that smoking at night (when the facility is short-staffed) is particularly dangerous.

Because smoking will likely be permitted in the building and some people will continue to smoke, rules for controlled smoking must be established. These rules should include the following:

- Absolutely no smoking is allowed in areas where oxygen or flammable liquids are in use, or in any other area marked "no smoking."
- Smoking by patients with psychiatric conditions that could make this activity particularly dangerous should be prohibited, restricted, or closely supervised, depending on the degree of the danger. However, the withdrawal of smoking privileges should not be used as a punishment.
- Smoking by patients confined to bed should be limited and supervised.
- Ambulatory patients should not be allowed to smoke in bed.
- Visitors must be apprised of and follow all smoking regulations.
- All outside contractors must also abide by facility smoking regulations.
- When smoking in a designated area:
  - Use only safety matches or mechanical lighters.
  - Crush all cigarette butts, killing the glow, and discard them in a safe place.
  - Do not dispose of cigarette butts in a wastebasket.

The CEO must ensure that all no-smoking areas are adequately demarcated using universal signs. The areas where smoking is permitted must be convenient for employees and patients to reach. This encourages smoking in designated areas. The trash receptacles and ashtrays in these areas must be of fire-resistant material, such as metal, and they should be emptied frequently. The room should be kept free of an accumulation of combustibles, such as papers and other rubbish, and should be regularly checked for smoldering cigarette butts, other fire hazards, and small fires. Finally, the room should contain appropriate portable extinguishers.

☐ Safety Considerations for Compressed Gas Cylinders

Health care facilities use a variety of compressed gases in everyday operation, including oxygen, nitrous oxide, and ethylene oxide. These gases, which are usually contained in pressurized cylinders, can be toxic and can support combustion or explosion. Because 100 percent ethylene oxide is highly flammable, many health care facilities are using 88/12 ethylene oxide, which is nonflammable.

In addition, because the gases are stored under extreme pressure, compressed gas cylinders must be handled with caution. The primary concern is protection of the valve assembly on the tank. Care must be taken to ensure that the tanks are properly secured to prevent them from accidentally tipping over, which could damage the valve assembly.

Valve assembly failure could result in an extremely dangerous condition called "rocketing," in which the cylinder is propelled with force enough to blast through a concrete wall—or a person. Consequently, it is imperative that the facility develop procedures for the safe handling, transporting, and storage of compressed gas cylinders. Some guidelines follow:

- Cylinders should be identified by labels or other means as to the gas contained. The label should also include appropriate warnings.
- Cylinders must have pressure-relief devices and connections that comply

with Compressed Gas Association standards.
- Valves must always remain closed on empty cylinders and cylinders that are not in use. When possible, valve protection caps should be used for added protection.
- If a defect appears on a compressed gas cylinder, or if it does not work correctly, never attempt to repair it yourself. Report any problems to the supplier.
- Compressed gas manifold systems that supply oxygen, nitrous oxide, or both to piping systems in the facility must be located in areas that can be secured from entry by unauthorized persons.

Storing Compressed Gas Cylinders

Cylinders must be stored:

- In designated areas only
- Away from radiators, direct rays of the sun, and other sources of heat
- In a well-protected, well-ventilated, dry location
- At least 20 feet from highly combustible materials such as oil and excelsior
- Away from elevators, stairs, or gangways
- Where there is no danger they will be knocked over or damaged by passing or falling objects, or subject to tampering by unauthorized persons

More specific storage restrictions include the following:

- Oxygen cylinders in storage must be separated from fuel-gas cylinders and combustible materials, especially oil or grease.
- Storage areas should be outside the building or in a room that is of one-hour fire-resistive construction. When the quantity exceeds 1,500 cubic feet, the room must be equipped with an automatic fire extinguishing system and be vented to the outside.
- Cylinders must never be allowed to stand alone because they may lose balance and tip over. All cylinders, whether full or empty, must be chained or secured in a proper tank cart.
- Full and empty cylinders must be stored separately. Empty cylinders should be labeled "MT" or "EMPTY."
- Empty cylinders must be returned immediately to the storage area.
- Smoking, striking of matches, and other open flames are prohibited in oxygen-enriched atmospheres and in oxygen storage areas.
- Cylinders should never be stored by laying them down or stacking them like cords of wood.
- Flammable and nonflammable cylinders must not be stored in the same area.
- Flammable gas storage areas should have explosion-proof electrical features.

Handling and Transporting Compressed Gas Cylinders

When moving cylinders, they must be treated gently. Never drag, drop, or roll cylinders or carry them over the shoulder. Use a cylinder cart or hand truck with the chain restraint in place. While transporting the cylinders, do not allow them to be struck or to strike each other because this may cause them to rupture. Do not use or handle leaking cylinders, but return them to the storage area and notify the supplier.

☐ Developing a Fire Plan

In addition to fire prevention tactics, the facility must also have an established means of responding in an orderly and safe manner to any fires that should occur. Health care facilities must have a way to protect helpless patients while guarding employee safety and minimizing property damage. These procedures and the fire safety program in general must be outlined in the facility fire plan. The Joint Commission requires that the plan address the fire safety needs of the entire facility and of specific areas. The plan must also discuss training for employees, staff, and volunteers.

To meet these and other requirements and to provide the highest level of protection, the fire plan must be uniquely tailored to the facility, its structure, and its personnel. However, the following guidelines are suggested for use as the general framework of an institution's fire plan. The plan should consist of two components—an immediate emergency response plan (for employees to remember and follow in the event of a fire) and a master plan.

Immediate Emergency Response Plan

This plan consists of a four-step procedure that employees should follow during a fire. This procedure should be memorized by all employees. The procedure recognizes that the best response to a fire in a health care facility is first, to sound the alarm, then to let others know there is a fire, then to combat the fire if possible, and finally, to evacuate, if necessary. It works best when expressed as an easily recalled acronym, such as *SAFE:*

1. *S—Sound* the alarm. Either pull it yourself or call out to someone else to pull it. Sounding the alarm is always the first step so that the fire department can be on its way while other activities are being performed. Because it is important to both sound the alarm and remove any person in immediate danger, employees should be encouraged to work together. One person can remove the patient, employee, or visitor from danger while calling out to another person to sound the alarm. But sounding the alarm is a priority.
2. *A—Alert* others. Quickly tell others in the area of the fire. Do this in a calm, firm manner. Do not cause a panic. Secure the area for the fire department. Close all doors and windows to prevent the spread of smoke and flames. Call the switchboard to give them verification and location of the fire. They may, in turn, make a follow-up call to the fire department.
3. *F—Fight* the fire. Do this only in the case of a manageable fire, one that you have training and experience to fight—for example, a fire in a wastebasket. If possible, two employees should fight the fire together, using two fire extinguishers. If you have any doubt about your ability to fight the fire, do not attempt to combat it.
4. *E—Evacuate* the area, if necessary.

With any immediate response, the actions are carried out through teamwork. This way, the steps of the response can occur simultaneously, allowing quicker control of the situation.

SAFE is just one of many acronyms that are used. Your facility may use a different one. The point of using such a formula is to ensure that employees will remember the steps to take, even under the strained emotional conditions evoked by a fire. It is wise to post the acronym throughout the facility. Even better, some facilities print the acronym on the back of employee name badges. The proper response, immediately carried out, can go a long way toward reducing damage and enhancing the master fire plan.

Master Fire Plan

The master fire plan deals with facilitywide and departmental fire safety. The first section of the master fire plan outlines fire protection measures such as those just discussed in the "Immediate Emergency Response Plan" section. The second section sets forth the response of the facility during a fire. Once the four-step immediate response has been carried out, the second phase of the master plan is activated:

1. The fire department is notified of the type and location of the fire with a follow-up call.
2. The fire page is announced over the public address system along with the location, repeated twice slowly and clearly.
3. Personnel whose services are vital to fire response gather in a preestablished location (often called the emergency control center), so that all decisions can be made centrally and collectively. Staff members to be included should be determined in advance and be named in the plan. They should include the administrator, safety personnel, engineering personnel, and so forth.
4. The administrator or designee assesses the progress and magnitude of the fire and keeps all departments apprised. This person also determines the need for patient evacuation.
5. All telephone calls and nonemergency pages are held. Incoming callers are instructed, "I am unable to complete your call at his time. Will you call again in a few minutes?"
6. A designated person is dispatched to meet the fire department at a designated entrance and to secure an elevator designated for their use.
7. When the danger has passed, instructions for giving the "All Clear" will be given by the person in charge.

Figure 7-3 (see p. 106) lists some departmental responsibilities during this time. However, this is not a comprehensive list, because each department should formulate its own plan.

□ Evacuation

Complete evacuation to the outside will rarely be necessary and is usually not the first step of an evacuation plan. However, in older buildings of highly combustible material and with leaky sprinkler systems, complete and early evacuation may be necessary. The need to continue vital patient care should be balanced against the degree of the immediate threat the fire poses to the area of the facility. The order to evacuate will come from the administrator or designee, in coordination with the fire department.

The evacuation may be partial or complete and may be accomplished in two ways:

- *Horizontal evacuation* describes the procedure of moving patients to a safe area on the same floor.
- *Vertical evacuation* refers to the use of stairs to move patients downward

to other floors or to the outside. Patients should never be evacuated to higher floors.

Patients, visitors, volunteers, and employees nearest the fire should be evacuated first. Ambulatory patients should be assembled, instructed to form a chain, and then moved in a group. Semiambulatory patients should be assisted one-on-one as they are pushed in wheelchairs or walk. Finally, bedridden patients may have to be carried. They can be wheeled in their beds but only in limited numbers, because this may block corridors. All patients should be given blankets to cover themselves during evacuation. Be sure to account for all patients against the patient card file once safety has been reached. Figure 7-4 (see p. 108) describes emergency patient carries. The evacuation plan should end by detailing procedures for recovery, such as how patients will be returned and what will be done with damaged areas.

□ Fire Brigade

The fire brigade is a group of specially trained personnel whom the administrator may appoint to respond to fires immediately, sound the alarm if it has not yet been pulled, and attempt to fight the fire. The fire brigade (if there is one) can act as an excellent fire protection resource. The brigade must consist of members from all shifts so that the facility is protected regardless of the time the fire occurs. A safety committee member should be designated team leader and should supervise and coordinate the response.

The fire brigade acts as a trained group that can respond promptly and adequately to manageable fires before the fire department arrives. Immediate action by skillful personnel can limit or even extinguish the fire in the time it takes for the fire department to arrive. The fire brigade's duties center on supplementing the immediate emergency response that staff members carry out. This includes removing patients and personnel from danger, using appropriate fire extinguishers, using other fire-fighting techniques (such as smothering the fire), and finding ways to work with the fire department.

There are two types of fires to which the brigade may respond—"incipient-stage fires" and "interior-structural fires." Incipient-stage fires are small, are limited to a well-defined area, and do not yet threaten the structure of the facility. Fire brigades must be thoroughly trained in fighting the type of fire for which they are designated. If they are only trained to fight more limited, incipient-stage blazes, they must know when to stop or when not to attempt to fight the fire at all. These groups must be trained in the use of appropriate fire extinguishers and in ways to protect themselves and to limit the spread of the fire.

Interior-structural fire brigades, on the other hand, must receive training equivalent to that a professional fire fighter receives, including use of hoses and respirators, rescuing of trapped individuals, and first aid. For health care facilities, this interior-structural type of brigade is rarely, if ever, used or necessary.

All fire brigade members, no matter what the type of brigade, must be completely familiar with the layout of the facility. Fire brigade training must be repeated at least annually. Finally, fire brigade members must be provided with appropriate personal protective clothing and equipment at no cost to them, and the employer must adequately maintain this equipment.

□ Fire Drills

A major component of fire safety training, and one that the plan must address, is fire drills. The Joint Commission requires that fire drills be conducted at least quarterly and include all personnel on all shifts. (The Commission recognizes real fires as drills as long as responses are documented and problems are addressed.) These drills may include facilitywide fire drills and those that are limited to a particular department. The drills can be preplanned, but occasional surprise drills are recommended to assess reactions to a situation more like a real fire. It is essential that all employees be involved, including second- and third-shift staff.

For a fire drill, employees should be taught these procedures:

1. Recognize the signal that means fire drill. Some facilities use a blinking lantern, marked flags, an announcement over the public address system, or personal notification of one or a few employees.
2. When this signal is encountered, respond to it as you would to an actual fire.
3. Rescue any persons in immediate danger. Dummies may be used for this purpose, and affected patients should be told what is occurring.
4. Confine the "fire" by closing all doors and windows.
5. Alert others. Pull the nearest fire alarm. The fire department should have been notified previously that a drill was to occur. Also telephone the switchboard, identify yourself, identify the location of the fire, and explain that it is a drill, unless the drill was preplanned and publicized.
6. Fight the fire. Locate the fire extinguisher and bring it back to the site. If the signs indicate a large fire or one you do not know how to fight, wait for the fire brigade or fire department to arrive.
7. The facility fire page will be transmitted on the public address system along with the location of the fire. Meanwhile, the administrator or designee will have been alerted to the "fire," and the fire brigade will have responded to the alarm by heading toward the fire.
8. Wait for more information or the order to evacuate.
9. When evacuating, follow master fire plan procedures for ambulatory, semiambulatory, and bedridden patients. Work rapidly but don't rush.
10. After evacuation, wait either for orders to evacuate further or for the "all clear."

Conducting quarterly drills is not enough. Their effectiveness must also be evaluated: Did the employee(s) who encountered the fire adhere to the immediate emergency response acronym used by the facility? Did the fire brigade respond promptly? Did designated personnel carry out their responsibilities correctly? Did everyone know what they were to do? Was evacuation speedy and orderly? Did alarm systems work correctly? Any fire protection equipment that did not function correctly should be repaired, and this action should be documented.

Employees should be questioned on how they viewed the drill and on ways for improvement. In the accreditation process, the Joint Commission will randomly sample employees, asking them to describe their role in the fire plan and to locate fire protection equipment and any equipment used to transport patients to safety. Some facilities time the evacuation or rate staff performance in the drill (including the performance of administrators) so that employees can see the evidence of improvement.

Finally, fire department personnel should be involved in the whole process. Sometimes, they even direct the drill or "spring" a surprise drill on the facility.

They must also participate in the evaluation of the drill. Methods to improve performance may be suggested and should be implemented by the facility. The facility should use all the resources available in the community, and the local fire protection district is among the most willing and helpful of these resources. Well-planned fire drills that are regularly evaluated provide the key to a rapid, orderly response during a real emergency.

☐ Conclusion

Much attention has focused on the many aspects of health care fire safety, such as codes, accreditation, detectors, fire department response, and the safety of the patient. Hospitalized patients have pressing concerns and must be able to assume that adequate consideration has been paid by health care personnel to the topic of fire safety. An effective fire protection program depends on all employees. Every employee should follow safe housekeeping practices with regard to preventing fires. Therefore, continuous training in work procedures, regular inspections of work areas, and close supervision of employee job performance are requisites for a successful fire prevention program.

Figure 7-1. Fire Extinguisher Classifications

Types of fire extinguishers in health care facilities correspond to three categories of fires. Each class of fire extinguisher should be used only on the kind of fire for which it was designed. For example, using a Class A extinguisher, which is meant for ordinary combustibles, on an electrical (Class C) fire can be extremely dangerous. All extinguishers must therefore be clearly labeled according to their classifications, and staff should be trained in recognizing and using the different types. Class ABC fire extinguishers can be used to fight all kinds of fires.

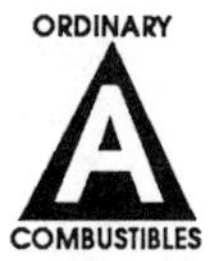

Class A. Class A fires involve ordinary combustible materials, such as wood, paper, cloth, rubber, and many plastics. Class A extinguishers rely on water-based solutions or dry chemicals, which are the most effective on this sort of fire. These extinguishers should be identified by a green triangle containing the letter A.

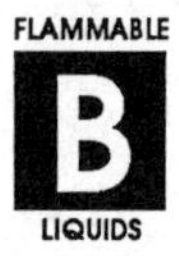

Class B. Class B fires involve flammable liquids, greases, oils, tars, oil-based paints, lacquers, and the like. With Class B fires, smothering the fire to interrupt the supply of air is most effective, so Class B extinguishers employ such substances as foam, dry chemical, or carbon dioxide. These extinguishers are labeled with a red square containing the letter B.

Class C. Class C fires are located in or near live electrical equipment. Here an extinguishing agent that will not conduct electricity is needed. Class C extinguishers, therefore, utilize carbon dioxide or dry chemical. These extinguishers are marked with a blue circle containing the letter C.

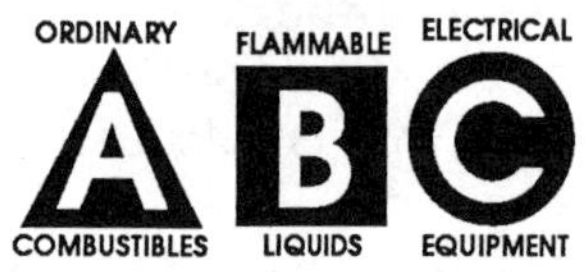

Class ABC. This type of fire extinguisher is capable of fighting Class A, B, or C fires. It can be useful to prevent confusion. However, ABC extinguishers may leave a sticky residue, so personnel in charge of fire safety may wish to choose Class B or C extinguishers for specific areas where these types of fires are more likely to occur. Multipurpose extinguishers are marked with the letters A, B, and C.

Figure 7-2. Fire Safety Inspection Checklist*

Sprinkler and Fire Detection System

______ Tested every 30 days by local fire department, unless other arrangements have been made.
______ Sprinkler system serviced annually by qualified agency.
______ Sprinkler valves accessible (with no recently stored material forming obstructions) and sealed open.
______ Sprinkler valves operate easily. No leaks, corrosion, or other defects noted in system.
______ Sprinkler water flow alarm tested.
______ Fire detection (alarm) system tested.

Fire-Alarm Facilities

______ Location signs in place.
______ Boxes unobstructed.
______ Date of last test: ______
______ Auxiliary boxes have sign indicating whether system is connected to fire department.

Fire Doors

______ Operative.
______ Unobstructed (no wedges to hold doors open).

Fire Hose (Standpipes)

______ Cabinet door operative.
______ Hose condition satisfactory (not rotted, wet, moldy, and so forth).
______ Nozzle in place; proper type.
______ Hose properly hung in rack; aired; rehung to avoid creases.

Fire Extinguishers

______ All extinguishers mounted in properly designated locations (refer to table 7-1).
______ Extinguisher seals intact and inspection tags properly initiated. To be inspected monthly, and serviced at least once a year.
______ Proper decals or other markings on extinguisher and wall to indicate type of fire on which extinguisher can be used.
______ No leaks, corrosion, or other defects noted.
______ Extinguishers unobstructed, ready for instant use.
______ No carbon tetrachloride or other vaporizing liquid used in any extinguisher.
______ Personnel informed on proper use.

Exits and Exitways

______ All exits clearly marked and exit lights on.
______ All exit lights clean and of proper wattage.
______ Exitways free from obstructions.
______ Furniture placed so that occupants can quickly and safely evacuate rooms.
______ Exterior grounds kept clear of objects that might impede evacuation of fire-fighting equipment.

Stairways

______ Doors at each level operate satisfactorily and are kept closed.
______ Stairways free of obstructions.
______ Landings properly lighted.

Fire Drills

______ Date of last fire drill: ______
______ All employees and staff members participate in drill.

Auxiliary Lighting

______ Auxiliary emergency generator operative: maintenance and operating condition.
______ Fire door properly maintained.
______ Lighting checked weekly; date of last test: ______

Careless Smoking Hazards

______ No smoking in bed a rule.
______ "No Smoking" signs placed where required.
______ Adequate supply of large-sized noncombustible ashtrays in every room, in lounge areas, and in other approved smoking areas.

Continued on next page

Figure 7-2. (Continued)

Electrical Wiring and Equipment

_____ All electrical equipment purchased and installed is tested for performance and safety.
_____ Appliances properly grounded.
_____ All motors of proper size; clean, free of lint; cords not frayed; grounded.
_____ Only qualified electricians are allowed to install or extend wiring.
_____ Use of extension cords discouraged. When their use is absolutely necessary, they should be checked to ensure they are not frayed or covered with grease or lint; length not over 10 feet; no multiple or "octopus" wiring connections to wall outlets; no cords under rugs or fabrics.
_____ All electrical circuits properly fused: 15 amp for general lighting circuits; 20 amp or more for special circuits.
_____ Emergency lighting system operable.
_____ Electric motors, fans, heaters, appliances, and fluorescent and other light fixtures free of combustibles; all such equipment easily accessible for replacement.

Heating, Ventilation, Flues, and Vents

_____ Natural fireplaces equipped with spark screens.
_____ Air-conditioning equipment filters clean.
_____ Heating plant checked and serviced by qualified agency (annually).
_____ Flues and vents free of dust and obstructions. (See **Kitchen.**)
_____ Fire door operating in boiler room and incinerator room.
_____ No combustible storage in room.

Housekeeping, Storage, and Waste Disposal

_____ Brooms, mops, rags, and other cleaning supplies stored properly in metal cabinets or approved cans.
_____ Paints, solvents, thinners, and other flammables stored in metal cabinet; oily rags in metal safety containers.
_____ Combustibles kept clear of stove, heating appliances, heating plant, and water heater.
_____ Dry leaves, shrubbery trimmings, and other combustibles kept away from buildings.
_____ No combustibles stored under stairways.

Kitchen

_____ Hoods, vents, fans, and ducts in good condition and free from grease.
_____ Hood filters cleaned regularly; date of last cleaning: _____
_____ Hoods equipped with appropriate automatic extinguishing devices.

Surgery and Obstetrics

_____ Monthly record readings of conductivity of surgery floor and furnishings, to check degree of insulation resistance.
_____ Amount of ether stored in surgery suite. (See **Alcohol, Ether, and Similar Chemicals.**)
_____ Proper relative humidity (R.H.) maintained; 50 percent R.H. if flammable inhalation anesthetics are used. Otherwise, it must be maintained according to the policy of the medical staff.
_____ Mechanical ventilation adequate.
_____ Equipment grounded, properly maintained, and tested periodically.
_____ Rubber tubes conductive in flammable anesthetizing locations.
_____ Rules and regulations posted.

Alcohol, Ether, and Similar Chemicals

_____ Properly stored.
_____ Properly dispensed.
_____ If refrigerator is used for storage of these chemicals, it is provided with explosionproof motor.
_____ "No Smoking" signs provided.

Compressed Gases (Nonflammable)

_____ Cylinders properly capped and stored in designated area.
_____ Cylinders properly secured by chain or strap to wall.
_____ Storeroom vented to outside.
_____ Fire door operative.
_____ "No Smoking" signs provided.

Figure 7-2. (Continued)

Miscellaneous Hazards

______ Nonsmoking areas equipped with adequate signs.
______ All curtains, draperies, and decorative fabrics in exitways treated with flame retardant.
______ Everyone in every department has been warned never to use flammable fluids for cleaning floors, clothes, or furnishings.
______ Gasoline is kept for use with power mower or generator; is properly located in safety can with self-closing cap.
______ Matches and cigarettes are taken from patients receiving oxygen. Relatives and visitors are warned about smoking and matches in restricted areas; members of the clergy are told not to light candles for religious rites.
______ Target areas such as mechanical equipment rooms, storage and supply rooms, and the laundry receive surveillance beyond routine checks for malfunctions and fire hazards.

*This inspection checklist is a guide. Items should be added or deleted in accordance with the size and operation of the particular facility. Each feature is to be checked monthly unless a different interval is indicated.

Figure 7-3. Fire Plan Responsibilities for Individual Departments

Nursing Units

Before a fire occurs:

1. One person on the 11 p.m.–7 a.m. shift should be assigned from each patient floor to act as a member of the fire brigade. Another should be assigned to secure a fire extinguisher at his or her location and be ready to respond, if necessary.
2. One person should be designated to turn on all corridor lights.
3. One person should be assigned to monitor the telephone to answer emergency calls or relay messages.
4. One person should be responsible for ensuring that all room doors are closed.
5. A list of patients should be convenient to see that all are accounted for.
6. Every nurse should become familiar with the facility fire plan.

In the event of a fire:

1. Carry out immediate emergency response.
2. Clear exits and elevator area. Do not allow elevators to be used.
3. If fire is in your area, ensure that all oxygen in operation is shut off in a safe manner. Oxygen shut-off valves are located ________. The (title) will make the decision as to when oxygen operation will be shut off.
4. If fire is not in the area, nursing managers should be prepared to use their personnel to care for patients transferred to the area or dispatch personnel to other areas.
5. Reassure patients who may become disturbed by the commotion.

Department Managers

Before a fire occurs:

1. Become familiar with the facility fire plan.
2. See that employees in their departments have been instructed as to their respective duties in case of fire.

In the event of a fire:

1. See that these duties are carried out.
2. Immediately upon hearing the alarm, ensure that all doors and windows in the area are closed.

Plant Services/Maintenance

Before a fire occurs:

1. Become familiar with the facility fire plan.
2. Designate appropriate personnel as members of the fire brigade.
3. Assign one person on the 7 a.m.–3 p.m. shift to meet the fire department at a designated entrance and secure a designated elevator at ground level for their use.

In the event of a fire:

1. Carry out immediate emergency response.
2. The director of maintenance will report to emergency control center, if a member of the emergency control group.
3. Regulate air-handling equipment.
4. Secure electrical room, boiler room, and other maintenance areas, as necessary.

Housekeeping

Before a fire occurs:

1. Become familiar with the facility fire plan.
2. The director of housekeeping will designate appropriate housekeeping personnel as fire brigade members.

Figure 7-3. (Continued)

In the event of a fire:

1. Carry out immediate emergency response.
2. All other housekeeping personnel remain in their work areas and assist when directed.
3. If necessary, help remove any patient to a safe area.
4. On the 3 p.m.–11 p.m. shift, one person will be assigned to meet the fire department at a designated area and secure a designated elevator for their use.

Dietary

1. Before a fire occurs, become familiar with the facility fire plan.

In the event of a fire:

1. Carry out immediate emergency response.
2. If fire or smoke is in the area, turn off gas and electrical machinery.
3. Personnel are to remain in the department.
4. If necessary, remove any person to a safe area.
5. Await instruction from emergency control center and be prepared to assist wherever needed.

Laundry

1. Before a fire occurs, become familiar with the facility fire plan.

In the event of fire:

1. Carry out immediate emergency response.
2. If fire or smoke is in the area, turn off machines.
3. Personnel are to remain in the department.
4. Await instructions from emergency control center (described in detail in chapter 8), and be prepared to assist wherever needed.

All Other Departments

1. Before a fire occurs, become familiar with the facility fire plan.

In the event of a fire:

1. Carry out immediate emergency response.
2. Personnel are to remain in their departments.
3. If necessary, remove any person to a safe area.
4. Await instructions from emergency control center and be prepared to assist wherever needed.

Figure 7-4. Patient Removal Methods

Infant and Child Removal

1. Place a blanket or sheet on the floor.
2. Place two infants in each bassinet, using diapers or small blankets for padding.
3. Place the bassinet in the middle of the blanket.
4. Fold the blanket over one end, fold the corners in, then roll the sides in to form a pocket.
5. Grasp the folded corners of the blanket and pull the infants to safety. Two persons (or, if necessary, one person) can drag eight babies to the prescribed area.
6. Alternatively, place as many children as possible in one crib, and pull the crib to the prescribed area.

Universal Carry

The universal carry is a method of removing a patient from a bed to the floor. It is a quick and effective method for removing a patient who is in immediate danger. This carry can be used by anyone regardless of the size of the patient.

1. Spread a blanket, sheet, or bedspread on the floor alongside the bed, placing one-third of it under the bed and leaving about 8 inches to extend beyond the patient's head.
2. Grasp the patient's ankles, and move the patient's legs until they fall at the knee over the edge of the bed.
3. Grasp each shoulder, slowly pulling the patient to a sitting position.
4. From the back, encircle the patient with your arms, place your arms under the patient's armpits, and lock your hands over the patient's chest.
5. Slide the patient slowly to the edge of the bed and lower him or her to the blanket. If the bed is high, instruct the patient to slide down one of your legs.
6. Taking care to protect the patient's head, gently lower the head and upper torso to the blanket and wrap the blanket around the patient.
7. At the patient's head, grip the blanket with both hands, one above each shoulder, holding the patient's head firmly in the 8 inches of blanket. Do not let the patient's head snap back.
8. Lift the patient to a half-sitting position, and pull the blanketed patient to safety.

Swing Carry

The swing carry requires two trained persons.

1. One carrier, feet together, slides an arm under the patient's neck and grasps the patient's far shoulder. The carrier's free hand is slipped under the patient's other upper arm, grasping it, and taking one step toward the foot of the bed, the carrier brings the patient to a sitting position.
2. The second carrier now grasps the patient's ankles, bringing the patient's legs at the knee over the edge of the bed.
3. Each carrier takes one of the patient's wrists and pulls it down over the carrier's shoulder, supporting the patient's body.
4. Each carrier reaches across the patient's back, placing one carrier's free hand on the other's shoulder.
5. Each carrier reaches under the patient's knees to lock hands with the other.
6. Standing close to the patient, the carriers bring their shoulders up and remove the patient from the bed, carrying the patient to a safe area.
7. At the safe area, each carrier drops on the knee closest to the patient, leans against the patient, and rests the patient's buttocks on the floor. The patient's torso is lowered to the floor, and the patient's head is placed on a pillow or like protection. The patient's head must always be carefully protected.

Blanket Drag

If vertical or downward evacuation by an interior stairway is necessary, in many cases one person can handle a helpless patient by using the blanket drag.

1. Double a blanket lengthwise, place it on the floor parallel and next to the bed, leaving 8 inches to extend above the patient's head.
2. Using cradle drop, kneel drop, or other suitable means, remove the patient from the bed to the folded blanket on the floor alongside the bed.
3. Grasping the blanket above the patient's head with both hands, drag the patient headfirst to the stairway.
4. Position yourself one, two, or three steps lower than the patient, depending on your height and the patient's height. The patient's lower body inclines upward.
5. Place your arms under the patient's arms and clasp your hands over the patient's chest.
6. Back slowly down the stairs, constantly maintaining close contact with the patient, keeping one leg against the patient's back.

Table 7-1. Departmental Guide for Fire Extinguisher Types and Locations[a,b]

Extinguisher Location	Most Likely Class of Fire	Recommended Extinguishers
All Areas		
Multipurpose (ABC) extinguishers are useful and practical for all types of hospital fires.		
Administrative Offices		
All areas	A, B, or C	Soda acid, water, or foam and CO_2 or dry chemical
Switchboard	A or C	Foam and CO_2
Accounting	A or C	Water and CO_2 or dry chemical
Admitting	A	Water
Purchasing	A	Water
Payroll	A	Water
Storeroom	A or B	Sprinkler system or water and CO_2 or dry chemical
Medical record room	A	Sprinkler system
Library	A	Sprinkler system
Housekeeping Department		
Storeroom	A or B	Sprinkler system or water and CO_2
Janitor closets	A or B	Soda acid and CO_2
Employee restrooms	A	Water
Employee locker room	A	Water
Doctors' lounge	A	Soda acid or water
Main lobby	A	Water
Engineering and Maintenance Department		
Boiler room	A, B, or C	Water or foam and CO_2 or dry chemical
Carpentry shop	A or C	Water or soda acid and CO_2 or dry chemical
Electrical shop	A or C	Foam and CO_2 or dry chemical
Paint shop	B	CO_2 or dry chemical
Elevator machine room	C	CO_2 or dry chemical
Elevator penthouse	C	CO_2 or dry chemical
Air-conditioning equipment room	C	CO_2 or dry chemical
Machine shop	C	CO_2 or dry chemical
Dietary and Food Service Department		
Main kitchen	A, B, or C	Water or soda acid and CO_2 or dry chemical
Dining rooms	A	Water or soda acid
Floor kitchens	A or C	Water or soda acid and CO_2 or dry chemical
Special-diet kitchens	A or C	Water or soda acid and CO_2 or dry chemical
Storerooms	A or B	Water or soda acid and CO_2 or dry chemical
Range hoods	B	Fusible link with CO_2 cartridge, steam vent, or dry chemical

Continued on next page

Table 7-1. (Continued)

Extinguisher Location	Most Likely Class of Fire	Recommended Extinguishers
Nursing Service		
Nurses' stations	A	Water or soda acid
Utility room	A or B	Foam
Solarium or lounge	A	Water or soda acid
Linen room/mattress room	A	Water
Treatment or examining room	A, B, or C	Water
Equipment storage room	B or C	Foam and CO_2 or dry chemical
Outpatient areas	A	Water
Central supply	A, B, or C	Water and CO_2 or dry chemical
Emergency department	A, B, or C	Water and CO_2 or dry chemical
Nursery	A or C	Water and CO_2
Formula room	A	Water
Nurses' room	A or C	Water and CO_2 or dry chemical
Auditorium	A	Soda acid or water
Classroom	A	Soda acid or water
Laundry Department		
Laundry workroom	A or B	Water and CO_2
Soiled linen room	A	Water or soda acid
Clean linen room	A	Water or soda acid
Sewing room	A or C	Water and CO_2
Central Service Department		
Central station	A	Water or soda acid
Equipment storage room	A, B, or C	Foam and CO_2 or dry chemical
Laboratory or Pathology Department		
Chemistry, bacteriology, serology, histology areas	A or B	Water and CO_2 or dry chemical
Basal metabolism room	A	Water
Electrocardiographic room	A or C	Foam and CO_2 or dry chemical
Morgue/museum room	A	Soda acid
Pharmacy		
General areas	A or B	Water and CO_2 or dry chemical
Alcohol storage	B	CO_2 or dry chemical
Radiology and Nuclear Medicine Departments		
Diagnostic room	A or C	Water and CO_2
Therapy room	A or C	Water and CO_2 or dry chemical
Viewing room	A or C	Water and CO_2 or dry chemical
Film storage room	A	Sprinkler system
Developing room	A	Water

Table 7-1. (Continued)

Extinguisher Location	Most Likely Class of Fire	Recommended Extinguishers
Surgical Suite		
Operating room	B or C	Foam and CO_2 or dry chemical
Anesthetic room	A or B	Sprinkler system inside; foam on outside of door
Delivery room	B or C	Foam and CO_2
Special Care Units (including intensive care units, intensive cardiac units, hyperbaric pressure chambers, and facilities for renal dialysis)		
Special machines, devices of electrical nature	C	CO_2 or dry chemical
Hyperbaric chamber with intensive use of oxygen	B	CO_2 or dry chemical or deluge system
Physical Therapy Department		
Physiotherapy	A or C	Water and CO_2
Occupational therapy	A	Soda acid or water

[a] CO_2 is carbon dioxide.

[b] All hospital personnel should know the fire hazards and locations of fire extinguishers within their own work areas. Some departments, such as maintenance shops, kitchens, and laboratories, are exposed to the hazards of several types of fires. Most departments, however, usually risk only one type. For example, most fires in administrative offices, rest rooms, and lobby areas have been the Class A type. The above extinguisher chart is arranged by department to help the safety surveillance team in comprehensive departmental inspections. However, it is intended only as a guide. Consult with local fire departments and insurance carriers to determine the specific needs of your facility.

Chapter 8
Emergency Preparedness

In the wake of a disaster, the community looks to the health care facility for assistance. Although the facility itself may have sustained significant damage, it must respond by continuing to serve the community with as little impairment as possible. This can only be achieved through comprehensive, coordinated planning. Staff members must know their assigned roles and perform them rapidly and efficiently, and the facility must work in tandem with other community agencies. A carefully prepared and successfully implemented disaster plan is the key to saving lives.

The facility must be prepared for excessive or unusual demands on its resources. An earthquake, for example, will not only result in an influx of critically injured persons but may prompt some to seek shelter and food at the facility. At the same time, the facility may still be reeling from internal disaster-related emergencies, such as building damage, fire, and power outage. An effective disaster plan prepares the facility for such multiple consequences while allocating resources to meet patient needs, continue service, and protect employees.

□ Identifying and Planning for Disasters

Identifying and planning for disasters requires the establishment of a group with emergency preparedness responsibilities. The chief executive officer, in cooperation with the safety director, appoints an emergency preparedness coordinator and a disaster committee. The committee can be small and is often a subsection of the safety committee. Representatives from departments that are vital in a disaster should serve as members, such as medical staff, nursing administrators, and personnel from the security, safety, engineering, and emergency medicine departments. The coordinator should be someone who is knowledgeable in disaster planning and who is motivated to serve the facility in this capacity. With one person directly responsible for emergency preparedness and a committee to support and assist that person, disaster planning gains direction and momentum.

Types of Disasters

The possible disasters are many, and their consequences are potentially devastating. The 1987 earthquake in southern California illustrates the results of poor planning. Although much time had been invested in ensuring that buildings were built to withstand such emergencies, health care facilities reported significant delays in implementing their disaster plans and inefficient action when they were implemented. Recent studies (Calandra, 1987, pp.13–14) have shown that earthquakes are almost as likely to occur in southern and midwestern areas of the United States as they are along the western coast. This highlights the need for planning at facilities nationwide.

Other disasters may have risks that are not as immediately evident as those of earthquakes—a chemical spill at a local industrial plant, a traffic accident involving a chemical spill from a truck or train, a multiple-car accident, a train collision or derailment, a plane crash, a bomb threat, or a power outage. As the use of radioactive agents proliferates in various industries, an accident involving the release of a radioactive substance at a business or during a train or traffic accident is increasingly probable. Therefore, facilities near nuclear power plants are no longer the only ones that need a plan for responding to a nuclear incident. Some familiar occurrences, such as a snowstorm or a thunderstorm, can spark an emergency situation both in the facility and in the community.

As a result, the emergency preparedness coordinator and committee must approach disaster planning with an open mind. They must consider all the possibilities and build flexibility into the plan so that the facility can respond to highly unlikely emergencies as rapidly and effectively as it responds to more foreseeable events. They must recognize the increasingly wide variety of disasters that are possible, as unfamiliar as they may seem. (Figure 8-1 on p. 121 provides a list of some possible disasters that could affect health care delivery.)

Location of the Facility

In identifying and planning for disasters, the coordinator and the committee have several factors to consider. One factor is the location of the facility, which has some bearing on the types of probable emergencies. Is the facility near the ocean, where hurricanes can develop? Is it in a part of the country that is predisposed to tornadoes, snow, drought, frequent thunderstorms? Does it border a body of water where boating and swimming accidents are likely? Is it close to mountains, resorts, or state parks where sporting accidents may occur? Each geographical location (part of the country, state, city) and terrain (mountains, water, forests) brings its own unique possibilities for disaster or emergency.

Proximity to other institutions and businesses can influence the type of disaster to expect. For example, if a hospital's catchment area includes an airport, planning for a plane crash will become a priority. If a facility is close to a train station, train tracks, or major highways, it must be prepared to deal with emergencies related to those types of transportation. Equally important to consider is the kind of business conducted in the community. Large manufacturing firms bring the increased possibility of a chemical release, a large-scale industrial accident, or a fire. The facility must be prepared with toxicological data and special treatment methods.

Resource Planning

Another major factor to investigate is the resources of the facility. Resources include space, supplies, equipment, and staff. The facility must know *beforehand* what its capabilities are, rather than scrambling to take an accounting after disaster strikes. The emergency preparedness coordinator and committee should take stock of the resources while they design the program.

Many questions should be asked. What equipment is available, and what will be done if it is damaged? How long would it be until necessary supplies ran out, and how would they be replaced? What staff services will be essential, and how fast can they be mobilized? How many beds could be made available, and how quickly? What kind of victims and how many of them could the facility accommodate? (For example, if the facility does not contain a burn unit, the plan should recognize that during a hotel fire in the area, many of the victims may have to be sent elsewhere.)

The emergency power generators must also be regularly started, tested, and maintained to ensure that the vital resource of electricity remains available. Do not assume that the generator will automatically work at peak efficiency during interruption of power. This assumption has often proved incorrect, and facilities have remained with limited or no electricity for weeks (sometimes months), greatly reducing the services the community so desperately needs in a disaster. Regular checks and maintenance can prevent such a frustrating and hazardous situation.

□ Utilizing Community Resources

Emergency preparedness is and must be a cooperative venture between the facility and the community. Without this coordination, the disaster effort becomes fragmented and dangerously unsuccessful. In both external and internal disasters, the community and the facility must be able to rely on a well-established cooperative relationship. During an internal disaster, the community helps the facility through fire fighting, law enforcement, and ambulance services. During an external emergency, the facility responds by providing on-site triage, information dissemination, treatment of victims, and even food and shelter. In disasters that impair both the facility and the community, the facility and the community rely on each other through a reciprocal relationship that benefits all involved.

This kind of coordinated effort does not occur unless a strong working partnership has been established prior to the emergency. Initiating and building on this relationship represents a major goal for emergency planning. A cooperative relationship with the fire department (as emphasized in chapter 7) is crucial because fire can and often does occur simultaneously with other disasters.

Because disasters affect all sectors of the community, there is often a body within local government that oversees emergency planning. Frequently called the Office of Emergency Services (OES), this agency is often operated under the local health department or other such office. The facility should include this organization in its disaster planning. The OES may be a source of information that can be used to develop a disaster plan. It can also assist in drills, in training, and in evaluation of the plan. Most important, the OES can help plan ways in which the facility can work with it and other community groups to speed disaster response and recovery.

The Superfund Amendments and Reauthorization Act (SARA) Title III, or "community right-to-know" act (discussed in chapters 2 and 6), is highly relevant to hospital emergency preparedness. Under Title III, hospitals near businesses that use large amounts of extremely hazardous chemicals must join a local emergency planning committee. Alternatively, if the hospital itself uses very large quantities of hazardous material, it may be required to serve on the committee as a generator. Whatever the case, the facilities involved in this planning should view their participation as an opportunity as well as a responsibility. Fire fighters, police, community officials, and the media also serve on the committee. By working closely with these individuals, the hospital can begin to establish a cooperative relationship with these groups that will be essential to a coordinated and efficient response during all types of emergencies.

As part of the communitywide cooperation, health care facilities must set aside their normally competitive stance toward each other. They should share disaster planning information and exchange disaster plans in an effort to work more efficiently with each other during a real community emergency. They may also cooperate in community disaster drills and help evaluate their own and each other's performance.

One of the most important aspects of this interaction between health care facilities is *mutual aid agreements.* These are formal, written assurances that each facility will provide well-defined services for the other in specific emergency situations. For example, if a disaster exceeds the bed capacity of one facility, it must be able to rely on another institution to take in victims. Mutual aid agreements should also be used to set forth the relationship between the facility and other groups, such as the emergency medical service, the police, and the Office of Emergency Services. The terms under which the support may be offered or received should be clearly spelled out, along with the type of assistance that will be provided, the estimated time the support will be necessary, and the way the agreement will be implemented. Each party should sign the agreement and include it as an appendix to its disaster plans.

Finally, there are many other sources of disaster planning information and assistance that the facility may want to contact. These include utility companies, to minimize the effect of an interruption in water, gas, telephone, or electrical service; the local Emergency Medical Services, for transportation of injured persons during an emergency; the National Disaster Medical System, which coordinates a national emergency preparedness program; the Federal Emergency Management Agency (FEMA), for emergency assistance and information; and the National Weather Service and the National Oceanic and Atmospheric Administration, for information and support in planning for natural disasters.

□ Writing an Umbrella Disaster Plan

Once the basic identification and planning have been accomplished, the emergency preparedness coordinator and committee turn their attention to writing the plan. There should be a master, or umbrella, plan that sets forth the foundation of the emergency response. After that is done, plans for specific internal and external emergencies are written. The Joint Commission on Accreditation of Healthcare Organizations (Joint Commission) requires brief, specific plans for evacuation; fires; bombs; interruption of electrical, gas, and water services; and other emergencies. Both the umbrella plan and targeted plans must be concise, readable, and easy to understand.

Some crucial components of the umbrella plan include the following:

- A system of command
- A control center
- Methods of communication

- A system for mobilizing personnel
- An organized process of patient management
- A public information system
- Disaster drills

Command

Command refers to an organized hierarchy of control that is enacted immediately following an emergency. The system of command determines who can declare an emergency, convene the control center personnel, and order evacuation. Usually the lines of succession begin with the administrator in charge. If this person is not available, the responsibility transfers to the emergency preparedness coordinator, then to the chief of the medical staff, and so forth. The chain of command, along with all other program elements, should take into consideration staffing shortages after normal working hours, on weekends and holidays, and at night. Having a system of command that is applicable in all situations prevents the anarchy sometimes associated with the early stages of a disaster and activates the organized emergency response.

Control Center

A *control center* must be designated. A control center is a place within the facility where decisions will be made. When an emergency situation arises, the administrator in charge goes there and summons the emergency control group. This group usually consists of the emergency preparedness coordinator or person responsible for disaster planning, the medical director, the director of nursing, the risk manager (or safety director), the director of maintenance or engineering (or both), and a public information manager. If these individuals are not available, or until they arrive, designated department representatives should take their place.

The emergency control group forms a team that monitors the progress of the emergency, authorizes emergency actions, coordinates activities with other community agencies, and activates mutual aid agreements. In essence, along with the administrator in charge, they control and coordinate the disaster response.

The room the control group uses should be identified in the plan, but it may need to be changed depending on the damage to the facility. It should be close to the center of activity but far enough away from any imminent hazards to maintain safety. The room should contain copies of the plan, pencils and pens, a typewriter, telephones and alternate communication systems, telephone directories, tables and chairs, a transistor radio, a coffee machine, and snacks, if possible. A room should be chosen that normally contains these items (such as an office), or these items should all be placed in the room *before* an emergency situation occurs. The command system and control center are perhaps the most important elements of the disaster plan, and they can be enacted in any type of emergency.

Communication

Communication is another vital component of disaster response. Cooperation within different areas of the facility and between the facility and the community is essential to a coordinated response. Switchboard personnel should be directed to keep all lines free except for emergency use, so that disaster information can get in and out. In many disasters, however, the telephone system will not be operational. The disaster plan *must* establish an alternate communication system. Shortwave radio may be used for external communication, and walkie-talkies can provide for interdepartment conversation. The control center and departments should be equipped with necessary communication devices in the event of such an emergency.

Mobilizing Personnel

Employees whose services are crucial to successful disaster response must be listed, and a *system for mobilizing them* should be outlined in the plan. These individuals include the following:

- Emergency department personnel, especially triage experts
- Engineering or maintenance personnel
- Nursing services personnel
- Medical staff, particularly any specialists in certain injuries that may be prevalent (burns, asphyxia, radiation sickness, and so forth)
- Security personnel
- Safety or risk management personnel
- Switchboard personnel (if the telephone system is still operational)

The plan should outline a system for contacting these individuals. The plan should contain the names, home telephone numbers, and pager numbers of all vital personnel. A telephone tree should be established, preferably using as callers persons who are not as vital to immediate response, such as support services staff. The plan should also prepare the facility to transport these personnel if conditions (snow, for example) make travel in personal vehicles difficult.

Patient Management

An organized process of *patient management* must be established. This includes procedures and paths of evacuation, criteria for relocating patients to other facilities if the building has been severely damaged, and a system of triage by which incoming patients are prioritized according to their injuries. The patient management element also controls when, how, and which patients are released to their families, if necessary.

Public Information

Public information is an important part of disaster response and one that is often overlooked. In many disasters, internal and external, the facility experiences a barrage of media attention. To ensure that all information being released is accurate, information must come from one source within the facility. For this reason, the emergency control group includes a public information manager. All staff members should be told not to answer any questions from the press but to refer them politely to this individual, explaining that he or she has more accurate and up-to-date information.

To prevent media personnel from interfering with the internal disaster response and to coordinate all information dissemination, an area should be designated as the public information center. This area should be close to the control center but, for obvious reasons, not the same room. This area should be comfortable and stocked with pencils and pens, a telephone, and perhaps a copier, snacks, and coffee. The public information manager should always remember that the way the media personnel are treated often influences their coverage.

Polite, respectful interactions with the media can enhance public perception of the facility's disaster efforts.

Drills

The plan must also delineate how staff members will be trained in executing the plan. *Disaster drills* represent one of the most effective ways to familiarize employees with the plan and allow them to practice their responsibilities. The Joint Commission requires facilities to carry out semiannual drills and to document and evaluate them. Scenarios should be as realistic as possible, and at least one drill a year should test response to an external emergency. All employees should be encouraged to contribute to the evaluation, as should community disaster agencies who participate. The Joint Commission may randomly question employees about the drill, including how it was evaluated. The entire disaster preparedness program must be thoroughly reviewed by the safety committee and updated each year or as facility capabilities or community needs change. All training, drills, and evaluations must be documented.

☐ Specific Plans for Some Common Disasters

Following are some tips for tailoring the facility's response to specific emergencies.

Bomb Threats

Unfortunately, today's society has seen an increase in bomb threats in virtually all public institutions, including health care facilities. One important step in dealing with a bomb threat is to have the person receiving the call listen carefully and get as much information as possible from and about the caller. Figure 8-2 (see p. 122) is an example of a form to be filled out by the person receiving the call. This form or a similar one should be conveniently located at switchboards and other phone locations.

Once the information has been gathered and the telephone call has ended, the person who received the call should notify his or her supervisor, who will inform the administrator. The administrator will then notify security and the local police. As necessary, the administrator will activate the emergency control group. Depending on state police protocol, searching should be initiated only with the help of the police. Searchers should be advised not to touch or move suspect objects. The search should be called off as the time of detonation nears. The administrator, with the help of the emergency control group, will give the order to evacuate.

Power Loss

The New York City blackout of 1977 illustrated the potential disaster caused by loss of electrical power. Although an outage in a health care facility cannot be compared to this citywide emergency, health care is dependent on electrically powered equipment, and a facilitywide power loss can take on disastrous proportions. A 1971 California earthquake caused service to be cut off to several hospitals. At least two patients died when life support was interrupted because emergency power generators failed.

Again, it must be emphasized that regular inspections, testing, and maintenance of the emergency power generator should be a priority. However, natural disasters may damage these as well. It is important, therefore, for the disaster plan to include arrangements for renting or buying new generators. The facility should have a clear understanding with the company that will supply the generator(s) so that the company can respond quickly to the facility's needs. The plan must also outline ways for the facility to continue operating with limited power.

Strikes

Although not usually disastrous, strikes can cause disruption in services and may lead to violence. Unlike other emergencies, there will be time to plan for a strike, for negotiations normally precede it. The administrator and the emergency preparedness personnel should make use of this time by planning how vital services will be continued, how nonstriking personnel can be reassigned, where temporary replacement personnel for support services can be found, and other ways to deal with a strike.

Computer Failure

Health care facilities have displayed a rapidly growing reliance on computers for many tasks (other than record storage), such as admitting, emergency department information gathering, patient monitoring, and security systems. Although computers contribute greatly to the efficiency of operations, an institution's dependence on them leaves it vulnerable to computer failure and even sabotage—both of which are potentially disastrous in a health care setting.

The facility should maintain an ongoing contract for the services of a repair firm (or firms) that agrees to respond immediately to any computer problems. The company should also be able to provide substitute equipment during lengthy repairs. This contractor or a qualified, experienced staff member should regularly inspect the system and conduct preventive maintenance. Equally important, computer storage drives should be "backed up" periodically, and the backup floppy diskettes, tape, or optical disks should be stored off-site. This reduces the possibility of losing months or years of data.

□ Conclusion

This chapter has emphasized the significance of planning to mitigate the effects of disaster. Emergency preparedness is a major responsibility for all health care facilities because they represent the guardians of health to the community and because the public looks to them for assistance and information in time of disaster. Potential types of emergencies must be identified in advance, and an effective umbrella plan, which can be tailored to the individual disaster, must be written. In addition, for disaster planning to succeed, it must be a coordinated community effort. With planning and practice, the facility can achieve a state of true *preparedness* that will enhance its response to and recovery from any type of disaster.

Figure 8-1. Potential Disasters That Could Affect Health Care Delivery

- Train accident
- Epidemic of food poisoning or other illness
- Nuclear accident
- Internal fire
- Fire in the community
- Chemical spill or release
- Airplane crash
- Multiple-car collision
- School bus wreck
- Bomb threat
- Terrorist attack
- Hostage situation
- Strikes, picketing, protests
- Power outage
- Utility (water, heat, natural gas) failure
- Computer failure
- Earthquake
- Monsoon
- Hurricane
- Tornado
- Blizzard
- Snowstorm
- Thunderstorm
- Drought
- Natural gas leak
- Building collapse
- Industrial or construction accident
- VIP disaster (for example, assassination or illness of a public figure)
- Flood

Figure 8-2. Sample Response to Bomb Threat Form

RESPONSE TO BOMB THREAT

If you receive a bomb threat, you may be able to reduce the hazards in a real situation.

Instructions:

1. BE CALM; BE COURTEOUS; LISTEN.
2. DO NOT INTERRUPT THE CALLER.

Date ______________ Time ___________ Person receiving call ___________

Exact WORDS of person placing the call: ______________________________

____

Questions to Ask:

1. When is the bomb going to explode? ____________________________
2. Where is the bomb right now? ________________________________
3. What kind of bomb is it? ___________________________________
4. What does it look like? ____________________________________
5. Why did you place the bomb? ________________________________

Try to determine the following:

Caller's Identity: ☐ Male ☐ Female ☐ Adult ☐ Juvenile Age ____

Caller's Voice: ☐ Loud ☐ Soft ☐ High ☐ Deep ☐ Raspy ☐ Pleasant

Caller's Accent: ☐ Local ☐ Not Local Foreign Region ______________

Caller's Speech: ☐ Fast ☐ Slow ☐ Distinct ☐ Disordered ☐ Stutter ☐ Slurred ☐ Lisp

Caller's Language: ☐ Excellent ☐ Good ☐ Fair ☐ Poor ☐ Foul ☐ Other

Caller's Manner: ☐ Calm ☐ Angry ☐ Rational ☐ Irrational ☐ Coherent ☐ Incoherent ☐ Deliberate ☐ Emotional ☐ Righteous ☐ Laughing ☐ Intoxicated ☐ Drugged

Background Noises: ☐ Office Machines ☐ Factory Machines ☐ Bedlam ☐ Train ☐ Music ☐ Quiet ☐ Voices ☐ Mixed ☐ Airplanes ☐ Party ☐ Street Traffic

Time Caller Hung Up: ______________________________________

Additional Information: ____________________________________

Action to take immediately after the call:

1. NOTIFY YOUR SUPERVISOR AND THE ADMINISTRATOR.
2. TALK TO NO ONE ABOUT THE CALL OTHER THAN INSTRUCTED BY YOUR SUPERVISOR.
3. BE PREPARED TO REPEAT SAME NOTIFICATION TO POLICE DEPARTMENT, AS REQUESTED.

Source: Reprinted, with permission, from National Safety Council. *Long Term Care Safety Management Manual: A Handbook for Practical Application.* Chicago: National Safety Council, 1987, p. 114.

Chapter 9

Incident Reporting and Investigation

Previous chapters described numerous ways to prevent incidents/accidents* through basic safety practices, including departmental safety, proper management of hazardous materials, and patient safety. Although a comprehensive safety program and rigorous risk-reduction measures will minimize incidents, they cannot prevent every untoward event from occurring. Once an incident does occur, it is up to the facility to follow up, determine what caused it, and take corrective measures.

Through a system of incident reporting and investigation, all incidents, even minor ones involving no injury or property damage, are taken seriously. They are viewed as symptoms of a larger problem—one that could cause other, more serious incidents if allowed to continue unchecked. These incidents are reported accurately and in a timely manner. They are then reviewed and action is taken to eliminate the causes and thereby prevent future similar incidents. What is achieved is the ability to learn from mistakes, which is crucial to the avoidance of future ones. In the process, injuries can be avoided, property damage can be minimized, and lives can even be saved.

□ Incident Reporting

The following sections describe benefits that can be gained by reporting *all* incidents that occur, discuss who should fill out incident reports, and list what information should be included in incident reports.

***Incidents* have been defined as unexpected, undesired happenings that have the potential to adversely affect the completion of a task or to cause injury or property damage. *Accidents* are the subsection of incidents that do result in injury or property damage, whether major or minor. In this chapter, we use the term *incident* as the broad category that includes accidents.

Which Incidents Should Be Reported?

All incidents should be reported, and they should be reported in a standard format. In many facilities, only the more severe injuries or accidents are reported. This is a mistake because less serious incidents often predict the occurrence of more damaging events. Incidents, sometimes called near-misses, should send out signals to staff that a situation that may cause an accident exists. For example, a visitor may complain at a nurses' station that the floor of the women's rest room is wet and slick in places. Although no injury or property damage has occurred, that potential exists. This type of complaint should be taken care of immediately. An incident report should then be completed and given to the risk manager or safety manager. As part of the data tracking system, the risk manager or safety director records the action taken. This information together with the incident report documents attests to the facility's concern for safety and willingness to improve hazardous conditions.

Prompt reporting of *all* incidents provides documentation of the measures the employer takes to protect the health and life of the facility's employees, patients, and visitors. This evidence may be necessary in several situations, such as Joint Commission on Accreditation of Healthcare Organizations (Joint Commission) reviews, workers' compensation procedures, state and local agency inspections, and inspections required by the Occupational Safety and Health Administration (OSHA). In some cases, incident reports may be used in defense of the facility in a court of law, should the incident spark criminal or civil proceedings. For these reasons, all incidents should be reported, regardless of whether injury or property damages resulted.

Another frequent, and possibly very expensive, mistake in health care incident reporting occurs when only safety-related incidents, such as falls or accidental injuries, are reported. Adverse outcomes of clinical care and actions during that care are often exempted from the incident reporting procedure. This amounts to a highly risky oversight (and one that could be expensive for the facility) because clinical incidents are those most likely to result in malpractice claims against both the clinician and the facility.

Documenting clinical incidents, which is often called "occurrence reporting," is usually a quality assurance function. Nevertheless, the safety department or director should work with the quality assurance personnel to set up a coordinated system, if none currently exists. This liaison should be a continuing one because clinical treatment and patient, employee, and visitor activities that are ancillary to patient care regularly intersect and have an impact on one another.

Who Should Report the Incident?

To some degree, the reporting system depends on the routine of the facility. Some organizations require supervisors to report the incidents in which their employees are involved. Although this does encourage involvement and concern on the part of supervisors, this system has several drawbacks. It removes the employee from a process that directly affects him or her. (The employee involved in the incident is the best person to know and describe exactly what happened.) In addition, having the supervisor fill out the incident report may make the report seem like a disciplinary action, and the employee may become reluctant to tell the whole story.

Having employees fill out their own incident reports, or at least allowing them to be involved in the process, gives them a sense of control over how the incident is viewed by management. It also eliminates the inaccuracies associated with communicating a story through a chain of people. Employee incident reporting can also be an excellent way to involve employees in safety. As they participate more fully in safety, they will begin to embrace the program's goals as their own.

A good incident reporting system requires the supervisor to review the incident and, when possible, discuss it with the employee. In this way, both supervisory and line employee involvement are maintained. Figure 9-1 (see p. 131) shows a flowchart of supervisory actions in response to employee injuries.

To ensure regular and appropriate reporting by all staff members, the facility must provide training and education in incident reporting techniques. All employees should receive training on when to file a report, how to fill it out, and whom to send it to. This is best accomplished using scenarios of real (or at least realistic) incidents. Using humor, imagination, and detail, such as fictional names and characteristics, can maintain interest. Chapter 10 describes training methods in more depth.

During training, the benefits of incident reporting to the employee should be enumerated, namely that the reports will be used to reduce hazards and prevent future incidents. It should be emphasized that, under ordinary circumstances, the reports will not be used against employees in any disciplinary action. Management should assure employees that action to prevent further incidents will be taken as a result of their reports. Finally, managers should be true to their word. Nothing motivates employees to participate in incident reporting more than the knowledge that their reports will get results.

What Should Be Reported?

There are probably as many incident report forms as there are facilities to report incidents. No one form can truly be considered ideal for every facility; the form depends to a large extent on the methods, style, needs, and preferences of the individual facility. However, there are some basic types of forms and some basic questions that all forms should ask in some way.

Two major types of form have emerged—the traditional narrative format and the checklist approach. The narrative format gives the writer more space to answer questions, elaborate, and individualize the occurrence. An example of this type of form is shown in figure 9-2 (see p. 132).

In the checklist approach, incidents are categorized—for example, "fall," "patient complaint"—and the appropriate box is checked off (see figure 9-3 on p. 134). This allows the computer to determine trends in types of incidents, times of day, shifts, and characteristics of personnel involved. Both forms have their virtues, although the trend is toward forms that are amenable to computer analysis. Checklists are acceptable as long as they provide room for narrative and for difficult-to-classify incidents and generally balance categorization with explanation.

Whatever form is used, it must be short and simple. The form should be no longer than the front and back of a page, should use questions that are easily understood, and should generally be as concise as possible while still eliciting the necessary facts. Some of the more important facts that any incident report form should be designed to obtain include the following:

1. *Who was involved in the incident?* This includes not just the full name but the age of the person and whether he or she is a patient, an employee, a volunteer, or a visitor. If the person is an employee, the person's job title, department, and date hired should be noted.
2. *Where did the incident occur?* This refers to the exact location. Be precise. Instead of "5th floor corridor," write "east hallway outside room

516" or "east hallway, 10 feet from nurses' station."

3. *When did the incident occur?* This requires the date, day of he week, exact time, and shift. This specific information aids in determining whether time of day, shift, and so forth increase the likelihood of this incident.
4. *What kind of incident occurred?* Either check the appropriate box or categorize the occurrence (for example, medication error, hazardous condition, theft, and so forth).
5. *What type of damage, if any, resulted from the incident?* First and foremost, were there any injuries? If so, describe them and note whether a physician was notified. Any property damage should also be discussed.
6. *How did the incident occur?* This is where a concise but informative narrative is required, one which details the events leading up to the incident. List any equipment or machinery involved, including the manufacturer, model number, and serial number. Explain also what work was being performed at the time of the incident.
7. *Why did the incident occur?* This is an important question, but one that can also create many problems. What is wanted here is *causation,* not blame. Incidents are almost *never* the result of a single cause, although there may be one "obvious" cause. For example, a patient almost received the incorrect medication but noticed that it did not look like his prescription. The chief cause of this incident was the nurse's mistake in taking out the wrong medicine container. However, many other factors may have contributed. The nurse may not have received adequate safety training, may have been rushed because the facility was understaffed, may have been unable to read a container with a defaced label, or may simply have been careless.

   Objectivity in determining causation is crucial. The supervisor should assist the employee in discovering causes. If management system deficiencies have contributed to the incident, they should be clearly identified and corrected. It does little good to pass all incidents off merely as results of carelessness or willful negligence on the part of the employee. Although these factors do play a part in some incidents, they are seldom the sole cause.
8. *What measures can be taken to correct these problems or remove factors that cause incidences?* Having those involved recommend action to be taken may provide excellent ideas that managers and supervisors may not have considered. However, not all incident reports ask for this information. Instead, corrective actions are sometimes elicited on separate follow-up forms.

After filling out the incident report form, the individual should sign and date it.

Routing

The chain of people through which the report is routed should be kept to a minimum. This way, confidentiality is maintained and, equally important, action is not delayed while the report is being reviewed. The first person to receive the report should be the employee's immediate supervisor, who may in some instances assist the employee in filling out the form.

In most cases, the incident report is passed on, preferably within 24 hours, to the safety director, risk manager, or other designated individual. This person reviews the incident and determines whether an investigation is necessary. The safety director or risk manager also decides whether anyone else needs to see the report, such as the administrator or the chief executive officer, employee health personnel, insurance representatives, the safety committee, or legal counsel. The number of persons within the facility who see the report should be limited. Distributing the report to numerous departments or individuals not only violates confidentiality and discourages future reporting but may also fragment the follow-up efforts. Photocopies of the report should be made at the discretion of the safety director or risk manager only.

☐ OSHA Reporting

Health care facilities fall within the Standard Industrial Code (SIC) under OSHA record-keeping requirements. The data from these records are used to compile factual information about accidents that have happened and to provide employers with a measure for evaluating the success of their safety program and identifying high-risk areas to which attention should be directed. The OSHA reporting is separate and distinct from any insurance or workers' compensation documentation. The major requirements focus on OSHA Form 200, OSHA Form 101, and the OSHA poster. These forms can be obtained from the Publications Office, U.S. Department of Labor, Third Street and Constitution Avenue, N.W., Washington, DC 20210.

Form 200, called the Log and Summary of Occupational Injuries and Illnesses, is used by organizations to compile their injury and illness statistics for each calendar year. It categorizes the incidents and furnishes room for detailed analysis. A copy of the totals and other specific information must be posted in the facility where such notices are customarily posted, from February 1 to March 1 of the following year.

Form 101 documents each "recordable" (a term defined in OSHA regulations) illness or injury. In this case, the facility's incident report form may be acceptable, assuming it documents at least the facts requested on Form 101. The information gathered on the facility's form must be maintained for at least five years.

Finally, the poster, which is provided by OSHA, describes the requirements of the 1970 Occupational Safety and Health Act (see figure 9-4 on p. 135). It must be posted permanently in a location where employees are most likely to see it.

☐ Techniques for Incident Investigation

Before embarking on investigations, it is important to be able to determine which incidents to investigate. Although a formal investigation of all incidents would be ideal, this goal is unrealistic. The safety director has many other responsibilities and may only attend to safety on a part-time basis. Moreover, as defined here, the number of incidents would far outstrip the capacity of safety personnel to investigate them all. One way to solve this dilemma is to begin with an informal investigation.

Informal Investigation

Informal investigations can be accomplished quickly and easily by the supervisor as he or she works with the employee to fill out the incident report. This type of investigation consists of an overview of the scene and a brief discussion with the employee and other persons involved. This can be done for every incident. The supervisor briefly notes the result of the investigation on a separate sheet, which is signed, dated, and forwarded with the report.

Formal Investigation

When a more in-depth inquiry is necessary, the safety director, safety staff, and, sometimes, members of the safety committee conduct a formal investigation. Knowing which incidents warrant investigation is a skill that can be developed with practice. It is not always true that only incidents resulting in severe injury or property damage should be investigated. Some near-miss incidents may suggest serious hazards that could cause a major accident and should therefore be investigated. In general, some conditions that suggest the need for formal investigation include:

- Patient or employee injuries
- A number of similar patient, employee, or visitor complaints
- A trend in time, place, or person involved in incidents
- A pattern of mishaps related to particular equipment or machinery
- A string of similar incident types
- Serious medication errors
- Adverse patient care outcomes
- Falls, even without injury
- Altercations involving physical contact between patients and staff

As many of these conditions suggest, patterns and trends are particularly significant and signal the need for a thorough investigation.

A formal investigation in many ways mirrors the supervisory informal investigation but on a larger scale. Surveying the scene, talking with those involved, and determining causation are the major elements. If a thorough incident report has been filled out, the investigators will have less work to do. Much of the information they are seeking deals with the who, what, when, where, and why answered by a well-designed incident report. They must also answer these questions:

- Who had the most control over the conditions surrounding the incident (for example, a supervisor, an employee, a manager)?
- What are the causes of the incident?
- What can be done to prevent recurrence?

It is important to remember, as previously mentioned, that incidents have many causes, including:

- Unsafe conditions, such as poor housekeeping and chemical hazards
- Unsafe acts, such as not following procedure or not wearing proper personal protective equipment
- Management system deficiencies, such as inadequate training, unrealistic procedures, or inadequate staffing levels
- Personal factors, such as tension, tiredness, or distractedness

These causes can influence each other. An employee may be tired (personal factor) because the facility is understaffed (management system deficiency). An employee may not use a safety guard on a power tool (unsafe act) because it malfunctions (unsafe condition). Investigators should realize that, more often than not, causes from each of these categories play a role in the incident.

It is also important to remember that time is an essential element in the investigation. The investigation must take place as soon as possible after the incident so that the facts are fresh in the minds of those involved.

Once the investigation has been completed, a report should be written. The report should describe both the methods and results of the investigation. Again, blame should be avoided; an objective discussion of causation will prove much more productive. Most important, the report should include corrective measures, ways to carry them out, and timetables for their implementation. The investigation report will serve as the working reference for the prevention methods introduced as a result of the investigation.

Developing Effective Interviewing Skills

One of the most effective investigation techniques is interviewing. The scene of the incident will provide clues as to what occurred and the conditions that may have contributed to the incident. The greatest source of information is the employee, patient, or other individual involved in the incident. The way to obtain the essential information from this person is through a personal interview.

Interviewing may seem deceptively simple: just ask a few casual questions and receive straightforward answers. Like most human interactions, however, interviewing is more complex. Interpersonal factors, fear of reprisal, and numerous other factors can affect the progress and outcome of the interview. In short, interviewing requires certain skills that can be developed through monitoring and practice.

To begin with, some attention should be paid to the place and time of the interview. The room should not create an atmosphere that is too formal. If possible, a place other than the interviewer's office should be chosen to help the employee understand that the interview is not a disciplinary action. The room should provide privacy, comfort, and freedom from distractions. Calls should be held and visits prevented.

The interviewer should start with some small talk to put the interviewee at ease and then say something like "Jeff," (or "Mr. Brown," whichever is appropriate to the relationship) "would you please describe for me in your own words exactly what happened?" The employee or patient should be allowed to tell his or her story, without interruption, before any questions are asked by the interviewer. This avoids influencing the employee's story with questions that lead in a certain direction (for example, "Why was there no label on the container?").

After the interviewee has told his or her story, the interviewer should repeat the story to ensure correct understanding. The interviewer may also want to have the employee pantomime any actions that may be difficult to describe. For example, the interviewer could ask, "Would you mind showing me how you turned to hear what your supervisor was shouting?" This may clarify any confusion.

After the employee's story has been told, there may be gaps or inconsistencies that remain. These will be the topic of the interviewer's follow-up questions. Again, never interrupt during the employee's first telling of the story.

One effective interviewing technique that should be used at this time is the open-ended question. Open-ended questions are those requiring more than a yes or no answer. Questions beginning in "how," "what," and "why" are often open-ended. For example, rather than asking "Did you tell your supervisor?" ask "What did you do next?" or "Describe what you thought then?" Open-ended questions allow the interviewee to answer fully, and they often provide a wealth of information.

In addition to asking the right kinds of questions, the interviewer should employ effective listening skills. Of the two elements of communication, speaking and listening, by far the one with which people most need practice is listening. One way to enhance listening is to clear the mind of all extraneous thoughts that do not relate to the matter at hand and concentrate on what the employee or patient is saying. To be sure that you have understood the speaker, you might repeat or paraphrase what he or she has said, as you understand it.

Pay attention to the emotional content of the speaker's words. People feel that they have been understood when the person they are talking to indicates he or she has registered the feelings and frustrations behind the words. Saying things such as "You seem upset," "I know you are worried," or "That must have been frightening" can go a long way toward showing sympathy and understanding. This emotional clarity will also provide clues to the logic and motivations of the person at the time of the incident, which is information that can be valuable in any investigation.

As the interview draws to a close, steer the conversation toward optimism about the future. The interview should always conclude on a positive note. Talk about the work that is being done to *prevent* such incidents from happening in the future. Thank the employee or patient for his or her assistance, and reiterate the concern of management and administration for employee and patient safety and health.

□ Data Tracking Systems

A comprehensive incident reporting system that is carried out routinely by the staff will probably generate voluminous amounts of information. However, the information, as such, provides no benefits. The success of incident reporting hinges on what is done with the information. Although individual incident reports may have some important uses, aggregate information is needed for the incident reporting system to meet its full potential.

Summary data from a number of incidents can uncover conditions difficult to detect even by monitoring every individual incident. For example, incidents that are months apart and in different departments may form part of a yearlong pattern that can be detected only with the record keeping and computation provided by an organized system of data tracking. Data tracking systems compile information on numerous variables involved in incidents, such as incident type, time of day, shift, and occupation. This way, trends and related factors become evident.

These systems do not have to be complex. A good log form such as that shown in figure 9-5 (see p. 136) keeps track of and compares many variables. This kind of form has space to note what corrective actions were taken and when, providing the ability to monitor the status of action taken on an incident. A good data tracking system allows the safety director, or person responsible, to keep track of follow-up on incidents and to ensure that action is taken and corrective measures are evaluated for effectiveness. In addition, OSHA Form 200 can be used or adapted for use in this capacity.

Many facilities are turning to computer programs rather than using forms. Often, these systems allow much more detailed analysis and streamline record keeping. When purchasing data tracking programs, the person responsible must ensure that support and training are available from the software company and that all necessary staff members are trained to use the system. This may require patiently overcoming computer phobia. If installing such software is feasible, the facility can reap many benefits. However, smaller facilities with fewer resources can have effective data tracking systems using regular documentation on well-designed forms.

☐ Conclusion

One of the most important elements of incident reporting is the way incident investigations are conducted. If the causes are not determined and removed, today's near-miss could result in tomorrow's serious injury. The purpose of incident investigation is to determine the facts, not to find blame. Effective investigations may include retracing the sequence of events, discovering multiple causes, and interviewing those involved. Incidents may have many causes, and it is important to find all of them in order to prevent accidents from recurring.

Figure 9-1. Supervisory Flowchart: Action Plan for Response to Employee Injuries

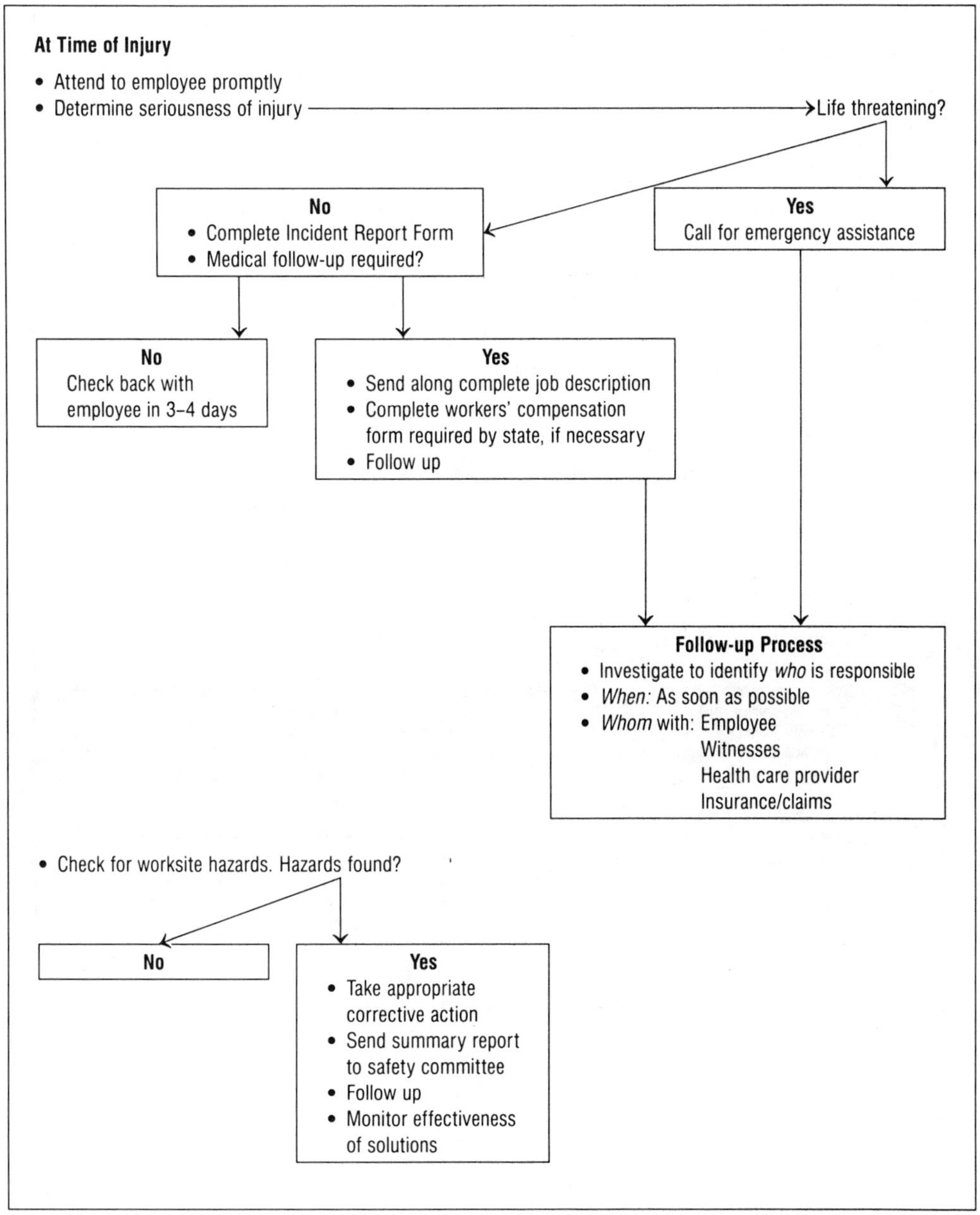

Source: Adapted from *Case Management of Employee Incidents,* published by Fred. S. James & Co. of Minnesota, Inc., 1986. Reprinted with permission.

Figure 9-2. Sample Incident Report: Narrative Format

cc Administration
Dept. Head
Safety Committee

James

CLAIM NO. ____________

SUPERVISOR'S REPORT OF EMPLOYEE INCIDENT

NOTE: This report is to be promptly and fully completed by employee's supervisor or designee except where noted. A response to all questions is required unless otherwise indicated.

Date of Incident ____________
Date Supv. Notified ____________
Date Report Completed ____________

_____ Near Miss _____ Medical Follow-up
_____ First Aid _____ Property Damage

WHO

Name ____________________ Age ______ Sex ______

Soc. Sec. No. ____________ Position ____________ Dept. ____________

Full/Part time (Circle) Permanent/Temporary (Circle)

Was employee engaged in usual work when incident occurred? (If not, specify position and date assigned): ____________

Names of other individuals involved: ____________

Witnesses: ____________

WHEN

Time __________ AM/PM Day: S M T W TH F SA Shift: First Second Third

WHERE

Location (identify precisely): ____________

HOW

Incident description (include specific description of employee's activities at time of incident): ____________

Identify physical/mechanical objects involved (tools, supplies, equipment, structures, etc. List mfg., model, and serial no.): ____________

Pre-existing disability/condition contributing to incident? (specify): ____________

Back Injuries ONLY: Were appropriate transfer techniques/lifting assists (transfer belt, patient lift, etc.) being utilized? (If YES, specify device): ____________

INCIDENT CAUSES (Check all that apply):

EQUIPMENT:
_____ Inappropriate for task
_____ Inadequate maintenance
_____ Inadequate design
_____ Other (MUST specify): ____________

PERSONAL:
_____ Failure to comply with established policies/procedures
_____ Failure to use appropriate equipment/techniques
_____ Lack of familiarity with task
_____ Improper motivation/attitude
_____ Other (MUST specify): ____________

ENVIRONMENTAL:
_____ Wet Surface
_____ Inadequate guards
_____ Fire hazard
_____ Congestion
_____ Electrical hazard
_____ Other (MUST specify): ____________

PROCEDURAL:
_____ Inadequate specification of equipment standards
_____ Inadequate specification of policies/procedures
_____ Inadequate communication of policies/procedures
_____ Inadequate enforcement of policies/procedures
_____ Other (MUST specify): ____________

Form 86-1 Rev. 9/86

Figure 9-2. (Continued)

WHAT

Describe nature and severity of injuries or property damage: ______

INCIDENT TYPES (Check all that apply):

____ Unexpected movement/sprain/strain	____ Chemical irritant	____ Struck by object/person
____ Fall from elevation	____ Puncture	____ Struck against object
____ Fall on level	____ Laceration	____ Caught between objects
____ Motor vehicle	____ Burn	____ Other (specify): ______

LOSS PREVENTION

Will employee lose work time as a result of the above? ______

What recommendations do you have to prevent a reoccurrence of this type of incident? ______

What actions are you taking or intend to take to prevent a reoccurrence of this type of incident? ______

Employee referred to: ____ Agency Clinic ____ EMS ____ Personal MD ____ Other (specify): ______

EMPLOYEE REVIEW

Above reviewed with employee; employee comments: ______

Employee Signature/Date

Supervisor Signature/Date

DEPARTMENT REVIEW

Does this work area have previous history of incidents? (If YES, indicate date of most recent incident and number of incidents in past 12 months): ______

Has above physical/mechanical object been involved in a previous incident? (If YES, indicate most recent incident and number of incidents in past 12 months): ______

Does this employee have previous history of incidents? (If YES, indicate date of most recent incident and number of incidents in the past 12 months): ______

Date employee hired: ______ Date filled current position: ______

Department Head comments: ______

Date First Report of Injury completed: ______ Date First Report forwarded to James: ______

Department Head Signature/Date

ADMINISTRATIVE REVIEW

Administration Comments: ______

Signature/Date

Source: Reprinted, with permission, from Fred. S. James & Co. of Minnesota, Inc., 1986.

Figure 9-3. Sample Incident Report: Checklist Format

An incident is any happening which is not consistent with the routine operation of the hospital or routine care of a particular patient. For each category mark as many items as are appropriate to adequately and completely describe the incident.

Hospital Attorney's Confidential Report of Incident (NOT PART OF MEDICAL RECORD)

FLOOR	UNIT	INCIDENT DATE	REPORT DATE	INCIDENT TIME	SHIFT
				____ A.M. ____ P.M.	____ 1st ____ 2nd ____ 3rd

PERSON INVOLVED	SEX	AGE	DIAGNOSIS
☐ 1 - Patient ☐ 2 - Visitor ☐ 3 - Employee ☐ 4 - Volunteer	☐ 1 - F ☐ 2 - M		

No. 20774

For Patient Incidents: List Patient's Full Name or Use Addressograph Plate
For Employee and Visitor Incidents: List Full Name and Address

PHYSICIAN'S STATEMENT

OFFICE USE ONLY

PRINT PHYSICIAN'S NAME

INCIDENT LOCATION

- ☐ 03 - CCU
- ☐ 09 - Corridors
- ☐ 11 - Delivery room (OB)
- ☐ 12 - Dietary
- ☐ 15 - Elevators
- ☐ 17 - Emergency room
- ☐ 18 - ICU
- ☐ 19 - Extended care/geriatrics
- ☐ 21 - Laboratory
- ☐ 23 - Labor room (OB)
- ☐ 24 - Laundry
- ☐ 27 - Nuclear medicine
- ☐ 29 - Nursery
- ☐ 31 - Nursing-medical
- ☐ 33 - Nursing-orthopedic
- ☐ 35 - Nursing-pediatrics
- ☐ 37 - Nursing-post partum
- ☐ 39 - Nursing-surgical
- ☐ 41 - Occupational therapy
- ☐ 43 - Outpatient/clinics
- ☐ 45 - Parking lots and sidewalks
- ☐ 47 - Patient's bathroom
- ☐ 49 - Patient's room
- ☐ 51 - Pharmacy
- ☐ 53 - Physical therapy
- ☐ 55 - Psychiatric unit
- ☐ 57 - Radiology
- ☐ 59 - Recovery (Post-Anesthesia)
- ☐ 61 - Respiratory therapy
- ☐ 63 - Shower room/bathroom
- ☐ 65 - Sitz bath
- ☐ 67 - Special care unit
- ☐ 69 - Surgery
- ☐ 71 - Stairs
- ☐ 73 - Visitor's lounge
- ☐ 75 - **Other** ____

INCIDENT TYPE - MEDICATION

- ☐ 18 - Administered without order
- ☐ 20 - Adverse medication reaction
- ☐ 22 - After discontinued
- ☐ 24 - Duplication
- ☐ 26 - I.V. Infiltration
- ☐ 28 - Medication on hold
- ☐ 30 - Medication theft/missing
- ☐ 32 - Omission
- ☐ 38 - Transfusion error
- ☐ 40 - Wrong dose
- ☐ 42 - Wrong medication
- ☐ 44 - Wrong rate
- ☐ 46 - Wrong route
- ☐ 47 - Wrong site
- ☐ 48 - Wrong time
- ☐ 50 - **Other** - ____

INCIDENT TYPE - MEDICAL

- ☐ 01 - Anesthesia service
- ☐ 02 - Emergency service
- ☐ 03 - Internal medicine
- ☐ 05 - Obstetrical service
- ☐ 06 - Physical medicine
- ☐ 07 - Radiology service
- ☐ 04 - Nuclear medicine
- ☐ 08 - Surgery
- ☐ 09 - Other

INCIDENT TYPE - FALLS

- ☐ 01 - Ambulating/with permission
- ☐ 02 - Ambulating/without permission
- ☐ 03 - Bed-rails up/restrained
- ☐ 04 - Bed-rails up/no restraints
- ☐ 06 - Bed-rails down/restrained
- ☐ 08 - Bed-rails down/no restraints
- ☐ 05 - Call light not used
- ☐ 10 - Chair or equipment/restrained
- ☐ 12 - Chair or equipment/no restraints
- ☐ 11 - Fainted
- ☐ 35 - Found on floor
- ☐ 07 - Improper footwear
- ☐ 13 - Incontinent
- ☐ 17 - Lost Balance/Dizzy
- ☐ 18 - Lowered side rail(s)
- ☐ 19 - Refused restraints
- ☐ 21 - Refused side rails
- ☐ 23 - Removed restraint(s)
- ☐ 29 - Unable to follow instructions
- ☐ 33 - Violated activity order
- ☐ 71 - Visitor assisted Pt. in ambulating without staff assistance
- ☐ 81 - **Other** - ____

INCIDENT TYPE - OTHER

- ☐ 52 - Assaults
- ☐ 56 - Broken/malfunctioning equipment
- ☐ 58 - Caught In/On/Between
- ☐ 60 - Contact with heat
- ☐ 62 - Diagnostic test at wrong time/sequence
- ☐ 64 - Needle stick
- ☐ 66 - Fire
- ☐ 71 - Consent
- ☐ 72 - Lost/damaged Pt./Visitor property
- ☐ 74 - Lost specimens
- ☐ 76 - Missing instrument(s)
- ☐ 78 - Missing needle(s)
- ☐ 80 - Missing sponge(s)
- ☐ 82 - Omitted diagnostic test
- ☐ 84 - Omitted treatment
- ☐ 86 - Patient escape
- ☐ 87 - Smoking
- ☐ 88 - Struck against
- ☐ 90 - Struck by
- ☐ 92 - Surgery check list not completed
- ☐ 94 - Wrong diet
- ☐ 95 - Wrong treatment/diagnostic test
- ☐ 96 - **Other** - ____

WAS PHYSICIAN NOTIFIED?
☐ YES ☐ NO

TIME NOTIFIED ____ A.M. ____ P.M.

NATURE OF INJURY

- ☐ 01 - Abrasion
- ☐ 03 - Aggravation of pre-existing condition
- ☐ 05 - Allergic Reaction
- ☐ 11 - Back
- ☐ 15 - Broken tooth/teeth
- ☐ 17 - Burns
- ☐ 21 - Contusion
- ☐ 23 - Deceased
- ☐ 25 - Fracture - Dislocation
- ☐ 27 - Head Injury
- ☐ 37 - Laceration
- ☐ 45 - Puncture
- ☐ 47 - Sprain/strain
- ☐ 50 - **X-Ray ordered**
- ☐ 41 - No Apparent Injury
- ☐ 51 - Not Applicable
- ☐ 49 - **Other** - ____

BRIEF DESCRIPTION OF INCIDENT: RECORD PATIENT'S CONDITION PRIOR TO INCIDENT; LIST WITNESSES: (Name, address, telephone - continue on reverse if necessary)

PRINT NAME AND PROFESSIONAL DESIGNATION OF PERSON COMPLETING REPORT

SUPERVISOR:

HOSPITAL COPY - USE REVERSE SIDE IF NECESSARY

OHIO 5/85
SPEEDIPLY• PAT D MCP• PAT D MBF 28

Source: Reprinted, with permission, from Wade, R. D. *Risk Management—HPL, Hospital Professional Liability Primer.* Columbus, OH: Ohio Insurance Company, 1983, pp. 88–89.

Figure 9-4. OSHA Poster

JOB SAFETY & HEALTH PROTECTION

The Occupational Safety and Health Act of 1970 provides job safety and health protection for workers by promoting safe and healthful working conditions throughout the Nation. Requirements of the Act include the following:

Employers

All employers must furnish to employees employment and a place of employment free from recognized hazards that are causing or are likely to cause death or serious harm to employees. Employers must comply with occupational safety and health standards issued under the Act.

Employees

Employees must comply with all occupational safety and health standards, rules, regulations and orders issued under the Act that apply to their own actions and conduct on the job.

The Occupational Safety and Health Administration (OSHA) of the U.S. Department of Labor has the primary responsibility for administering the Act. OSHA issues occupational safety and health standards, and its Compliance Safety and Health Officers conduct jobsite inspections to help ensure compliance with the Act.

Inspection

The Act requires that a representative of the employer and a representative authorized by the employees be given an opportunity to accompany the OSHA inspector for the purpose of aiding the inspection.

Where there is no authorized employee representative, the OSHA Compliance Officer must consult with a reasonable number of employees concerning safety and health conditions in the workplace.

Complaint

Employees or their representatives have the right to file a complaint with the nearest OSHA office requesting an inspection if they believe unsafe or unhealthful conditions exist in their workplace. OSHA will withhold, on request, names of employees complaining.

The Act provides that employees may not be discharged or discriminated against in any way for filing safety and health complaints or for otherwise exercising their rights under the Act.

Employees who believe they have been discriminated against may file a complaint with their nearest OSHA office within 30 days of the alleged discrimination.

Citation

If upon inspection OSHA believes an employer has violated the Act, a citation alleging such violations will be issued to the employer. Each citation will specify a time period within which the alleged violation must be corrected.

The OSHA citation must be prominently displayed at or near the place of alleged violation for three days, or until it is corrected, whichever is later, to warn employees of dangers that may exist there.

Proposed Penalty

The Act provides for mandatory penalties against employers of up to $1,000 for each serious violation and for optional penalties of up to $1,000 for each nonserious violation. Penalties of up to $1,000 per day may be proposed for failure to correct violations within the proposed time period. Also, any employer who willfully or repeatedly violates the Act may be assessed penalties of up to $10,000 for each such violation.

Criminal penalties are also provided for in the Act. Any willful violation resulting in death of an employee, upon conviction, is punishable by a fine of not more than $10,000, or by imprisonment for not more than six months, or by both. Conviction of an employer after a first conviction doubles these maximum penalties.

Voluntary Activity

While providing penalties for violations, the Act also encourages efforts by labor and management, before an OSHA inspection, to reduce workplace hazards voluntarily and to develop and improve safety and health programs in all workplaces and industries. OSHA's Voluntary Protection Programs recognize outstanding efforts of this nature.

Such voluntary action should initially focus on the identification and elimination of hazards that could cause death, injury, or illness to employees and supervisors. There are many public and private organizations that can provide information and assistance in this effort, if requested. Also, your local OSHA office can provide considerable help and advice on solving safety and health problems or can refer you to other sources for help such as training.

Consultation

Free consultative assistance, without citation or penalty, is available to employers, on request, through OSHA supported programs in most State departments of labor or health.

More Information

Additional information and copies of the Act, specific OSHA safety and health standards, and other applicable regulations may be obtained from your employer or from the nearest OSHA Regional Office in the following locations:

Atlanta, Georgia
Boston, Massachusetts
Chicago, Illinois
Dallas, Texas
Denver, Colorado
Kansas City, Missouri
New York, New York
Philadelphia, Pennsylvania
San Francisco, California
Seattle, Washington

Telephone numbers for these offices, and additional area office locations, are listed in the telephone directory under the United States Department of Labor in the United States Government listing.

Washington, D.C.
1985
OSHA 2203

William E. Brock, Secretary of Labor

U.S. Department of Labor
Occupational Safety and Health Administration

Under provisions of Title 29, Code of Federal Regulations, Part 1903.2(a)(1) employers must post this notice (or a facsimile) in a conspicuous place where notices to employees are customarily posted.

Figure 9-5. Sample Data Tracking Form

Date and Person Reporting	Safety Issue Present Circumstances/Contributing Factors	Desired Circumstances	Suggested Solution(s) Action/Responsible Party(s)/ Implementation Date

Figure 9-5. (Continued)

Results of Action	Satisfactory? Yes or No	Further Recommended Action(s) Action/Responsible Party(s)/ Implementation Date	Review Date	Results of Action	Satisfactory? Yes or No

Source: Reprinted, with permission, from National Safety Council. *Long Term Care Safety Management Manual: A Handbook for Practical Application.* Chicago: National Safety Council, 1987, p. 105.

Chapter 10
Training and Development

In discussions of safety, one word appears more frequently than any other—training. Few if any other elements of safety can be considered as crucial to the success of a safety program as ongoing training in safe attitudes and practices. Regulatory and voluntary compliance agency requirements should be enough in themselves to warrant a full-fledged safety training system. Virtually every major law and regulation affecting health care calls for staff education to ensure that employees understand what is required of them and their employer.

For some standards, training is the essential element, as in the Hazard Communication Standard, which mandates that the worker has a "right to *know*"—to be *informed* and *trained.* Regulatory emphasis on training reflects the belief among compliance organizations that facility-sponsored continuing education is the most effective way to ensure that their requirements are met.

Even without this emphasis by the Joint Commission on Accreditation of Healthcare Organizations, the Occupational Safety and Health Administration, the Environmental Protection Agency, and numerous other agencies, training would still be intrinsic to the successful operation of a health care facility. As with every learned skill, constant practice and access to instruction represent the only means of ensuring continued capability and expertise in the use of safety techniques. Employees must be helped to understand the need for safety, the concepts underlying program elements, and the techniques of risk avoidance.

Because of its significance, safety training must draw on careful planning and attention to quality. The ability to conduct effective, enjoyable training is, without a doubt, a skill—and one that can be developed. This entire chapter is therefore devoted to training and development—not only to emphasize the importance of training but to provide practical guidelines for successful training.

□ Developing a Safety Training Program

Before launching an extensive safety training program, those individuals responsible for it should devote some time to planning. During the planning phase, efforts should be made to integrate safety education with all other training. Safety then becomes a part of not only every job requirement but of all job training. The benefit of this integrated approach is that it presents safety as an element of the employee's job performance, which will be viewed as such by management.

A Step-by-Step Approach

Planning successful safety training requires an organized step-by-step process. Some elementary steps in planning and evaluating training include the following:

1. *Determine training needs.* There are certain topics that should be included in all health care safety training—infectious disease hazards, fire prevention, incident reporting, disaster preparedness, hazardous waste disposal, electrical safety, and body mechanics, to name but a few. Many of them may already be part of the facility's training through various departments or in-service education. Such tools as testing, direct observation of performance, and questionnaires can be useful in identifying the facility's specific training needs. In addition, items such as incident reports and statistics on employee injuries can determine the need for education on body mechanics or correct needle disposal. The facility's needs provide the raw data from which the training program will be developed. Deciding what training needs exist also depends on the unique characteristics of the facility staff. Factors such as average age, educational background, area of the country, and previous experience all have a bearing on how much and what type of training is necessary. Training for an older, more experienced staff must focus on performance upgrading that avoids condescension. Safety training for a largely younger staff or for employees in a new facility will start with the basics.
2. *Determine facility capabilities.* Once training needs have been outlined, those responsible for safety programs must determine how the facility can fulfill these needs. Staff members of health care facilities have widely varying personal and educational backgrounds. This diversity provides a pool of people with different talents and abilities, which often can be used in safety training. Outgoing, involved individuals may be chosen as instructors. Creative employees may help to write program materials or design audiovisual materials. Technical experts can review content. Many health care facilities find that using these staff resources greatly enhances the quality of training and the participation of employees.

   Not every facility can or should undertake all training in-house. There are innumerable outside resources, and not all are costly. Consultants may design and instruct in-service education. Associations to which the facility belongs may provide materials or assistance. Relatively inexpensive written training programs are available to minimize development time and cost. Whatever the resources of the facility, high-quality, cost-effective training is feasible.
3. *Assign training responsibilities.* In order to ensure an organized program, someone should be designated to coordinate all safety training. This person should possess both interest and experience in training and in safety. He or she must be capable of working with other departments. It would be preferable if this person would coordinate all training programs in the institution. This encourages greater integration of safety and job training.

In addition to the appointment of an overall training coordinator, individuals should be chosen for other aspects of training. On the basis of staff resources (identified when determining facility capabilities), individuals should be chosen to be course instructors, help to write and develop programs, plan room arrangements, and conduct the other necessary tasks in planning and implementing safety training.

4. *Design the program.* Once these steps have been accomplished, it will be relatively easy to design and prioritize training, that is, how the learning needs will be met (audiovisual aids, study guides, lectures), who the instructor or presenter will be, and how to determine when the needs have been met (testing, observing, feedback).
5. *Carry out the training.* At this time, attention to detail is important. Seating should be arranged to facilitate interaction. The room—chairs, air temperature, noise level—should be comfortable and conducive to learning. Breaks and, where the session is long or includes a meal hour, refreshments should be provided.
6. *Evaluate the training and revise it accordingly.* The success and effectiveness of the educational session should be determined so that future training can better meet staff needs. Many techniques can be used to determine what employees learned and what they liked and disliked about the program. Using techniques such as giving tests before and after the program, providing evaluation forms, and monitoring employee practices after the training can be helpful. A model evaluation form appears in figure 10-1 (see p. 146).

Content of a Safety Training Program

Although each facility will have its own unique needs and priorities, some basic components should be included in any safety training program:

- Explanation of the facility's safety program—components, staff, resources, and so forth
- Explanations of pertinent regulations and how to comply
- Hazardous and infectious materials handling
- Accident prevention techniques, such as back-injury prevention and electrical safety precautions
- Fire protection methods
- Patient safety
- Disaster preparedness
- Use of personal protective equipment
- Accident reporting
- Information on resources available to employees, such as the safety committee and Material Safety Data Sheets
- Infection control precautions, including AIDS/hepatitis B virus (HBV) protection

These represent minimum safety training topics. Others chosen will depend on the needs of the facility, the problems experienced, and state and local regulations.

In planning and implementing practical safety training, it should be recognized that different positions in the health care hierarchy require distinct approaches. The three levels of training that should be treated separately are orientation for the new employee, employee training, and management training.

☐ Orientation for the New Employee

The emphasis on safety begins during the employee's first contacts with the organization—hiring and orientation. Chapter 1 discussed hiring safety-conscious employees, which is a key step to ensuring safe practices at all levels of experience. Another way is through a program of new employee orientation.

It is the desire of all new employees to feel accepted. Trainers can respond to that desire during orientation. By gathering all new employees together, the trainer helps each beginner feel less conspicuous. Supervisors and other trainers should welcome the recruits in a friendly and personal way. They should emphasize that safety is a major part of the philosophy and everyday operation of the facility. Safe actions can be presented as a way to "fit in," and participation in safety programs can be presented as one method of becoming an established member of the facility's team.

Orientation must cover many topics in order to serve its purpose of welcoming employees and helping them come up to the facility's standards. There are a multitude of questions in the minds of new employees, especially about terms of employment. Sick days, vacation, benefits, and other vital information should be imparted early in the orientation. With these questions answered, new employees will feel more at ease and be open to absorbing other information.

Orientation safety training should include an introduction to each of the minimum elements of safety. This way, the groundwork is laid not only for safe practices early in the employee's term of service but for later safety training as well. The introduction must remain general in order to allow for time to cover each topic. Informal training on the job, as well as later in-service training, will fill in details.

Finally, orientation represents the ideal time for upper-level management to demonstrate its support. Top management and administrators can do this by attending the safety orientation part of the program. They should reiterate the welcome that other personnel have extended and emphasize the significance of safe job performance. This shows employees that what they have been told about the importance of safety is true. At the same time, upper-level administrators can briefly outline management's efforts, such as the safety program and incentives, to protect the health and safety of the facility's most valuable resource—its employees.

☐ Employee Training

Although new employee orientation is designed to introduce and underscore the significance of the overall safety program, regular employee in-services or educational courses will explain how these measures are actually carried out. The emphasis in ongoing employee training is on skills—developing and reinforcing the procedures that form the foundation of the safety program.

Skills training differs from routine information dissemination in that the teaching of skills is less didactic and passive. Skills training requires interaction and two-way communication rather than just lectures. The trainer must first explain the reasons for methods and their benefits. In helping an employee actually learn the skill, participation on the part of the employee is crucial. A step-by-step method for employee training is often effective:

1. *Discuss the policy underlying a procedure.* For example, the instructor could explain that accident prevention is a prominent part of the safety program. Because incident reporting can be used to prevent future acci-

dents, incident reporting methods must be taught to all employees. The reason for learning a skill, and how that skill will help employees, is important to establish at the outset.

2. *Give employees the information they will need to undertake the procedure.* In the case of incident reporting, for instance, the instructor would distribute and explain the report form used by the facility and discuss reportable occurrences.
3. *Explain the steps of the process.* Breaking the skill into manageable steps assists in comprehension.
4. *Demonstrate the skill.* For incident reporting, the instructor could discuss an incident scenario and show (on an overhead transparency) how it would be reported.
5. *Repeat the demonstration, but with feedback.* The instructor could ask employees, "What would I do next?" "What should I write here?"
6. *Supervise practice.* With the example of incident reporting, employees could be divided into groups and given a case study or scenario to react to as if it had happened to them. The instructor would facilitate interaction but remain unobtrusive at this stage.
7. *Discuss and review.* The instructor could discuss the case and reports that have been filled out. Questions, comments, and suggestions should be encouraged. With employee input, the reasoning behind actions and the steps involved in the procedures could be reviewed. Instructors should hand out evaluation forms and revise the training program as necessary.
8. *Document all training in personnel files.* Documentation is important for proof of compliance and staff competence.

This step-by-step process requires trainers to explain what will be taught, to teach it, and to review what was learned. It emphasizes learning a skill and understanding the philosophy behind it. Finally, this process allows for interaction and employee input, elements that have been shown to increase the probability that new skills will be used in everyday job performance.

□ Management Training

Training those who will manage employees requires a carefully designed approach. Management training will center less on developing skills than on helping others to cultivate them. Because of their crucial role in ensuring that safety practices are followed, managers must be taught, in short, how to train.

This "train-the-trainer" approach consists of a number of elements. As with employee training, conceptual information comes first. Important concepts to cover include the origin of the safety program, the reasons for it, the need for each element, and management's role in the program's effective operation. This explanation of program philosophy should go deeper than the similar discussion in employee training.

Although it is important to demonstrate the benefits to the manager, it is of equal importance to emphasize the program's benefits to the entire facility. Safety should be tied to the mission of the facility and to the formal performance evaluation system.

Supervisors and managers need not be instructors in the formal safety program to be considered trainers. Their routine management responsibilities, it should be explained, require constant training of employees. Each time they demonstrate a technique or praise or rebuke an employee, they are involved in training. As a result, managers wield the most control over what employees learn to do. Managers should realize during training that this influence can be used to teach and encourage safe procedures, which will protect the employee, the department, and the facility as a whole.

Although managers may be pleased by the importance of their role, they may also feel inadequate as trainers, particularly if trainers' responsibilities include formal classroom instruction. For this reason, and to enhance the quality of the training employees undergo, managers should receive instruction in training methods, including public speaking, communication, and techniques to enliven the training process. Helpful hints for beginning trainers/teachers are listed in figure 10-2 (see p. 147).

It may not be possible to accomplish all this in in-service training or other in-house instruction. Therefore, professional development of managers should be encouraged through outside conferences, seminars, and so forth. Many associations and professional groups offer courses for continuing education credit. The investment will pay off when supervisors and managers can conduct effective and enjoyable training, minimizing the need for outside speakers and reducing the overall cost of high-quality training. Finally, as with all other instruction, management training should be evaluated and documented.

☐ Working Successfully with Other Departments

Just as integrating safety into other training is essential to establishing the importance of safety, so is cooperation among departments. The safety department, or other responsible department, cannot act alone in developing and implementing safety training. Often, the resulting program will be viewed by employees as something unrelated to them and unnecessary. Without departmental interaction, individual departments' safety training needs are often not met.

Consequently, safety trainers should consult with all departments in designing safety training. The safety director can meet with the nursing administrator, for example, and ask for his or her input. What are nursing's safety training priorities? What do nursing personnel see as vital to the protection of the facility? The safety director can invite the nursing administrator (and other department managers) to participate in program development, such as teaching the medication error session, writing the AIDS/HBV protection lesson, and so forth. Often, just this brief discussion and an invitation to assist in training will generate commitment among other departments to the safety training program.

Those with safety training responsibilities should also work with department managers and employees to design targeted training sessions. These in-service sessions are geared toward solving specific problems that have been identified in a department, such as a rash of patient falls or hazardous chemical spills. When managers and employees in departments see that safety training can benefit them by solving their individual problems, their commitment and participation in facilitywide training will grow. It is then that safety training can become an effective and adaptive force for the protection of employees and the facility.

☐ Training Methods and Strategies

During each of the preceding levels of training, instructors use some type of training method, knowingly or not. In many cases, the "strategy" will be as simple as a classroom lecture. Whereas this teaching method is an effective one with which employees feel comfortable, trainers should be aware of the wide array of other techniques available for the enhancement of learning. Also, the lecture has several disadvantages when used alone and may be entirely inappropriate for some learning situations and audience needs.

The following describe a few commonly used training techniques that can boost the success of in-services and other training:

- *Discussion.* The instructor facilitates discussion with and among the students. Discussion is useful to encourage participatory learning and to gather ideas and solve problems creatively.
- *Demonstration/skills training.* The instructor acts out steps to be learned, repeating the procedure with learner input. An example of this strategy is the step-by-step technique outlined in the employee training section. This is quite effective in teaching a skill.
- *Role-playing.* During role-playing, the instructor assigns parts for participants to play. Often, the circumstances for the role-playing are scenarios that test what has been learned. For example, in an in-service session on interviewing skills for accident investigators, one student could play an injured patient and another the safety director. This reinforces learning and allows students to understand the real-life roles of other personnel in the facility.
- *Brainstorming.* Like discussion, brainstorming relies on verbal interaction. All group members are allowed to suggest any ideas that come to mind, however odd or irrelevant. Brainstorming often generates many valuable options during problem solving.
- *Case study.* The case study approach consists of reading (or viewing on a videotape) a realistic situation and responding to it. For example, a disaster involving a tornado, several hundred community casualties, and loss of electricity could be described. Employees from different departments would then explain step-by-step what they would do in this case. This method has wide applicability, such as in teaching incident reporting, emergency preparedness, and hazardous chemicals procedures.
- *Self-study.* This method uses programmed lessons and exercises, which the student studies alone. The instructor then follows up with group discussion and perhaps reinforcement testing. Self-study allows all students to progress at their own pace. However, students must be motivated to do lessons on their own.

These represent a very few of the major training strategies. Others include audiovisual materials (audiotapes, videotapes, overhead transparencies, charts), learning games, questioning, class exercises, listening tests, and handouts. The number and type of techniques possible are limited only by the trainer's imagination.

Some factors will influence the training methods used. For example, cost differs for various techniques. Advanced audiovisual materials, such as interactive video, for example, will cost more than an informal group discussion. Similarly, having a year of in-services designed and instructed by a consultant may involve more expense than one interactive video.

Drawing on staff ingenuity, some training needs can be creatively filled in-house. For example, some facilities have written and directed their own training videos, often with great success. Although they are not always of the highest quality, the videos are enjoyed and understood more by employees, who can relate to topics acted out by people they know in the facility where they work.

Another factor influencing training methods is the audience. The trainer must always consider the characteristics (background, age, education) of his or her audience and gear training to suit those traits. For instance, self-study may not be effective when employees are not motivated to work on their own, and role-playing and other games have limited applicability with adults, who may consider them childish. Guidelines for selecting a teaching method are outlined in figure 10-3 (see p. 147).

The point is not to be too conservative in choosing training techniques but at the same time to target the approach to the audience. The appropriate use of inventive training strategies not only increases the volume of what is learned and later practiced, but makes training a much more enjoyable experience for everyone involved—even the reluctant trainer.

☐ Conclusion

Safety training is one of the more positive actions that can be taken in health care facilities. The effects of the training efforts become readily apparent and can be measured. The training process can become a positive tool for the evaluation of the safety program. Good training produces skilled and productive workers, as well as safe workers.

Figure 10-1. Sample Training Evaluation Form

1. Topic and date of in-service: ______
2. Overall rating of in-service (1–10: 1 = worst; 10 = best): ______
3. Rating of instructor (1–10) in the following categories:
   Preparation ______
   Content of presentation ______
   Speaking ability ______
   Responsiveness to audience ______
   Other (please list) ______
4. What did you like *most* about the in-service?
5. What did you like *least* about the in-service? ______
6. What information did you find most valuable? ______
7. Do you have any suggestions for changes or improvements, or any other comments? Please list (use back of form if necessary). ______
8. Please list your department. ______
9. What departmental issues or other topics would you like to see covered in future in-services? ______

Thank you for taking the time to fill out this form. If any of your concerns cannot be addressed using this form, feel free to discuss them with the instructors and (person responsible for the training). We value your opinion, and your comments and suggestions will be used in designing future training and educational programs.

Sincerely,

(Signature of person responsible for the training)

Figure 10-2. Helpful Hints for Beginning Trainers

- **Flexibility** is important in the classroom. Students may become excited about an issue or portion of content. Allow for discussion even though the issues may not be part of the lesson plan or don't cover specific objectives. Individuals may be stimulated to research further information and become involved in further sessions.
- **Variety** may be introduced by providing for a number of different activities. Learners remain alert and become responsive when there is an exciting and stimulating environment in the classroom.
- Provide for some **personal time** for each learner.
- Offer **approval,** a nod, a smile for good work done.
- Student **self-evaluations** are often helpful. A positive approach should be used and an outline given. Items such as: "What have you learned and in what areas have you achieved success?" and "In what areas do you need more assistance?" are items which need to be explored.
- Provide for **eye contact.** Look at each student many times. Faces which demonstrate a frown, preoccupied look, or panic in taking notes offer a strong clue that some students are lost in the learning process.
- Ask for student **assistance** and **analysis** as to what went on in the classroom. Did you break the monotony or specific train of thought by using an audiovisual aid? How did the group respond?
- **Participative learning** gets adults actively involved in the teaching–learning process.
- **Answer** all questions asked. Adults must not hesitate to ask questions by thinking that perhaps the questions are not good ones or that their peers have the answers.

Source: Reprinted, with permission, from Dyche, J. *Educational Program Development for Employees in Health Care Agencies.* Los Angeles: Tri-Oak Educational Division, 1982, p. 51.

Figure 10-3. Guidelines for Selecting a Teaching Method

- Determine facility resources—staff, funds, time.
- Decide which options will fit within budget restrictions.
- Determine the appropriate method for the audience.
- Match the technique to training needs. For example, skills training requires hands-on learning, but explaining a new regulation may only require lecture and discussion.
- Apply new teaching methods gradually and with explanation, especially for groups accustomed to lecture only.
- Choose only those techniques with which you, the trainer, are comfortable. If you feel awkward or inadequate using a specific method, avoid it until your experience level allows you to feel more comfortable with the strategy. When you are having difficulty, the students will perceive it and may take your instruction less seriously.
- Use only the audiovisual materials that relate to the topic at hand. Avoid the use of films or videotapes as entertainment only. Provide ample time before and after any audiovisual aid to discuss it, and help the audience integrate the material. The audiovisual aid should seldom, if ever, be the focus of the entire training period.
- Preview all audiovisual materials and read all written training materials before discussing them with the class.
- Learn from mistakes and bad choices of training methods, using student evaluation forms.

Chapter 11

Special Considerations in Mental Health Settings

As risks to general acute care hospitals have escalated throughout the past few decades, a parallel and less widely recognized crisis was developing in mental health facilities. Growing public sophistication and scrutiny has increasingly questioned the efficacy of psychiatric treatment modalities, the competence of staff, and the extent of abuse in mental health settings. The media have boosted awareness through reports of abuse, understaffed facilities, and invasive treatment (for example, electroconvulsive therapy or administration of psychotropic medication). Films and television have brought to light the past wrongs of the fields of psychiatry and psychology, as witnessed by the popularity of movies exposing notorious cases.

The courts have upheld negligence and malpractice claims for failure to prevent suicide, homicide, and violence by and against present and former patients. Mental health institutions of all kinds have found themselves the target of tightening regulatory controls in the areas of safety and quality of care.

These risks cannot be treated in the same manner as comparable ones in a general hospital. The staff of a mental health facility or unit must often juggle conflicting obligations—to the individual patient, other patients, staff, and the community. They must gauge such critical and subjective qualities as suicidal tendencies, possibility for outward aggression, and unwillingness to cooperate in treatment.

They are also responsible for designing effective treatment plans that protect the patient and others from harm, while avoiding infringement on basic patient rights. Finally, the staff finds itself in the position of determining when it is ethical, judicious, and legal to subjugate patient desires or rights in order to protect others or for the long-term good of the patient. As a result of these unique pressures and demands, a distinct approach to safety in the mental health setting is required. As part of this approach, certain high-priority needs should be emphasized.

☐ Preventing Patient Abuse

Among the high-priority needs of mental health facilities is the prevention of patient abuse, the phenomenon most often attracting the glare of publicity and malpractice. As a result of underreporting, reliable statistics on psychiatric patient abuse are unavailable. However, it is clear that the unique characteristics of the patient population and staff in the mental health setting aggravate staff/patient tension. Patients may be confused, severely disabled, aggressive, and even violent and may exhibit bizarre behavior. These individuals live in close quarters with what are often some of health care's least trained and most underpaid staff, such as aides and orderlies. In some facilities, the majority of routine care is dispensed by these employees.

The combination of these factors—the characteristics of patients, poorly trained and underpaid staff, and supervision by low-level employees—can prove volatile. Staff members with meager training may fail to understand that destructive actions by patients do not represent a personal affront. Employees may be frustrated with their jobs and vent this anger at patients. They may not know how to deal constructively with patient aggression. Procedures may not be in place for preventing situations that may provoke patients. What results are incidents ranging from mildly insulting remarks to shouting at patients, threatening, hitting, biting, scratching, rape, and even, on occasion, wrongful death.

Patient abuse is one of the major safety, liability, and patient care problems for the mental health facility or unit. Much the same situation exists in long-term care facilities for the developmentally disabled. One of the most effective ways of dealing with the phenomenon of abuse is by training staff to respond properly to angry or destructive patient behavior. A comprehensive policy on preventing abuse, reacting to violent outbursts, and reporting and investigating abuse must be written and in place. This document should not be filed away and never used, but should serve as a guide in training and in monitoring staff performance.

Dealing with Agitated Patients

Employees should know that anger progresses through more or less recognizable stages, so many times being alert to body language or other clues can provide a head start in dealing with an agitated patient. The first stage often manifests itself in *irritation* or *jumpy* behavior. The patient may do something unusual for him or her, such as snapping at other patients or staff. The patient may withdraw, mutter, or fidget. Often, this early stage of anger is characterized by tense posture and restlessness.

At this time, the employee should try to understand the patient's situation. Many times, the patient is acting in response to a legitimate source of stress. The employee should talk in a soothing (although not condescending) manner. The employee should be instructed never to be confrontational but to attempt to reason with and reassure the patient. If possible, the staff member should remove or dispel the source of anxiety.

If these measures are unsuccessful, the patient may advance to the next stage of anger, often called *aggravation*. In this stage, behavioral clues become more pronounced. Body tension deepens; hands and teeth are clenched. The patient may curse or, as in the case of paranoid individuals, rant about bizarre or imagined threats. Employees should never take any threats lightly, even—and perhaps especially—from those expressing delusions of persecution or the desire to commit a violent act. The importance of not reacting to aggression as a personal attack cannot be overemphasized. This is key to helping employees minimize their anger and their need to strike back.

At this time, employees should continue to attempt verbal intervention. However, the tone of the employee's words may become more authoritative (while still nonthreatening). The employee should say that he or she would like to help but that destructive behavior will not be tolerated. The employee should offer again to discuss the problem privately. While the patient is in this stage of anger, the employee should take special care not to seem intimidating. Do not "corner" the patient; leave her or him an avenue of escape. Avoid sudden movements and remain at least 10 feet away from the patient.

Finally, the stages of anger culminate in actual *rage*, the stage in which physical violence is possible. This is the point at which gentle physical management by staff may be necessary. It is crucial that staff members be taught established methods of physically restraining or transporting violent or potentially destructive patients. They should follow a well-defined procedure for bed restraints, as outlined in chapter 5.

□ Guidelines for Physical Management

In cases of advanced anger and aggression, the facility has a duty to protect the patient, the staff, and other patients from harm. For this reason, the patient may need to be forcibly removed from the situation and detained in a "control" or "holding" room or in another adequately protected room. Before transporting the patient, the employee should ask the patient to go willingly himself or herself or to accompany the employee peaceably. Many incidents of physical management might have been avoided if this step had not been neglected. Angry or upset patients may feel that they have been attacked if they are not aware of the option to go willingly.

When it appears that physical management will be necessary, the employee should call for help. Often a code (such as "Dr. Armstrong") is preferable to avoid exciting the patient and onlookers. Proper physical management should be carried out by at least three staff members to avoid injury to staff or the patient.

Now is not the time for explaining what to do. Employees should have been trained in safe physical management procedures so that they can carry them out on short notice. One employee, either the one most involved in the incident or the one who is most experienced, should announce the type of physical management and assign each employee a part of the body. The employee might say, "All right, we will use the basic control hold procedure. I've got the torso; John, you take the head; and Cathy, you get his feet."

The staff member in charge should say comforting things to the patient, explaining what is being done and why. The employee might say, "We are going to remove (restrain) you so that you won't hurt yourself or others. You'll be all right. We want to help you because we're concerned about you." If possible, a gentle pat on the back or other kind gesture sometimes calms the patient. Staff members should not admonish the patient with the threat of punishment.

Once the patient is restrained, all potentially dangerous items should be removed from the patient's person or pockets (such as combs, belts, pens, knives, and necklaces and other jewelry). After the patient has been escorted or carried to the appropriate room, an employee should inform the patient when he or she will be allowed to leave. Checks should be made frequently, and staff should be aware that destructiveness may turn inward at this point, making suicide possible. The patient should *never* be left in the room longer than the established period of time. All actions, including checks, should be fully documented, and an incident report should be filed. All incidents in which patients or staff are injured should be investigated, and changes in procedures and training should be made accordingly.

☐ Patient Rights

In mental health settings (as well as in long-term care facilities), it is essential to guard the rights of those who may have difficulty doing so themselves. This is particularly true of patients committed to an institution, who have already lost some of their rights as citizens. Just because a patient has been committed to an institution or has consented to care does not invalidate the responsibility of caregivers to consult with the patient whenever possible and uphold other basic rights. To be sure that this takes place, many states and localities have instituted standards requiring health care personnel to guard certain patient rights. These rights may differ from region to region, so each facility is urged to contact the appropriate agency in its area for guidance in these matters.

One of the major patient rights issues that has emerged in these settings is the application of so-called "intrusive" or "invasive" therapies against the will of the patient or for punishment. According to the Joint Commission on Accreditation of Healthcare Organizations (Joint Commission), special justification must be provided for at least the following modalities:

- Electroconvulsive therapy (ECT)
- Seclusion
- Restraints
- The administration of psychotropic medications
- Psychosurgery or other surgical procedures to alter or intervene in an emotional, mental, or behavioral disorder
- Behavioral modification procedures that use aversive conditioning
- Other treatment procedures for children and adolescents, such as restriction of privileges, and so forth

These require justification and caution in use because of their effects, the way in which they work, and their potential for violating patient rights. Cases have occurred in which, for example, ECT was used repeatedly as a punishment or to mollify destructive or troublesome behavior.

Although these practices have, for the most part, been extinguished, the public, the courts, and patients remain particularly sensitive to ECT. Before initiating ECT for a child or an adolescent, the Joint Commission requires that two qualified child psychiatrists who have training or experience in the treatment of children and adolescents, and who are not directly involved in the treatment of the patient, follow this procedure:

1. Examine the patient.
2. Consult with the psychiatrists responsible for the patient.
3. Document in the patient's medical record their concurrence with the decision to administer such therapy.

Although this procedure pertains only to children and adolescents, a similar procedure is recommended for the administration of this therapy and other highly controversial therapies to adults as well. Another invasive procedure has attracted widespread attention and concern. Often called chemical management, this is the practice of administering psychotropic medications where not demonstrably indicated by the patient's condition, or merely to pacify the patient.

The facility should develop and implement policies and procedures dealing with controversial treatment methods and patient refusal of treatment. These policies should recognize the right of patients to refuse treatment and outline a step-by-step procedure that will take place as a result of the refusal.

When a patient has refused a treatment method, the attending physician should discuss with the patient and the patient's family the reasons for refusal and try to convince the patient of the value of the method. If this fails to alter the patient's stance, the physician should discuss alternatives with the patient's treatment team, documenting both discussions. Seeking an impartial consultant's opinion can increase the justification for either applying or withholding the treatment.

The psychiatric administrator may be called in to interview the patient, the patient's family, the physician, the consultant, and members of the treatment team and make a final decision. This appeals process will ensure that no one person makes an executive decision to override patient wishes and will provide greater justification for the course finally taken. Once the decision has been reached, through proper channels, to administer psychotropic medication, the patient's condition must be periodically reassessed. Doses and frequency of administration may need to be reduced as progress becomes evident. This is true for cases of patient *cooperation* as well as refusal.

All of the steps taken to formalize the facility's response to patient refusal of a treatment procedure must be fully documented. Although this documentation may seem burdensome, it represents one of the most effective ways that treatment staff can protect themselves and the facility from liability. (See figure 11-1 on p. 158 for a list of patient rights in mental health and long-term care facilities.)

☐ Suicide Precautions

Just as general health care institutions are being held accountable for outcomes of medical/surgical treatment, mental health facilities have been found liable for negligence in the suicide deaths of patients under their care. Extended further, this responsibility has been applied to violent patient behavior outside the facility (that is, once the patient has left the facility), especially when it can be shown that staff members had reason to believe that the patient could be dangerous. This poses a major challenge to the mental health facility—to adequately assess and respond to the threat of patients to themselves and others.

Psychiatric patients first require careful assessment and later monitoring. A patient who may not display evidence of suicidal or aggressive ideation on admission may develop these tendencies later in his or her stay. Policies and procedures must describe assessment and monitoring criteria for determining potentially dangerous behavior. The policy must include, at a minimum, the following:

- *Discussion of the capabilities of the facility to adequately care for and protect the facility from dangerous patients.* In many mental health units within general care hospitals, structural security and trained staff members will not be sufficient to protect personnel, patients, and the community. These facilities should outline procedures for transferring patients to an appropriate facility, when necessary.
- *A set of criteria for determining dangerousness upon admission and regularly thereafter.* Indicators of dangerousness include but are not limited to:
  - Previous assaults or destructive behavior
  - Threats of violence or suicide
  - Chaotic family life
  - History of abuse or abusiveness
  - Hostile feelings
  - Severe environmental stressors
- *A provision for closely monitoring suicidal or destructive patients.*

- *Procedures for when a patient will be transferred to a designated control or holding room, and a description of how this room should be maintained.* The room should contain no items that could be used as weapons, including plastic trashcan liners and glass mirrors, or shower heads or rods that can support body weight.
- *Directions for checking the patient very often, at least every 15 minutes.* The checks should be adequately documented. The patient should also be provided with regular meals, access to a toilet, and opportunities to bathe.
- *Provisions for maintaining a patient committed to a control or holding room.* His or her belongings will be checked for any items that could be used for self-injury; the patient will be given plastic utensils with meals; and all straps and ties will be removed from the patient's clothing.
- *Specification that a time-limited order for seclusion or restraint will be written by a physician within 12 hours after the initial use of the measure.*
- *Discussion of how the patient and family will be kept advised at all times of progress and treatment.*
- *Requirement that the patient's progress in seclusion be regularly monitored so that the patient can rejoin the group at the earliest opportunity.*
- *Direction never to exceed time limits for seclusion.*
- *Requirement that the order to seclude be reviewed and, if renewed, be reissued and signed by the attending physician every 24 hours.*
- *Procedure requiring that all suicides and attempted suicides be documented in an incident report and be investigated.*

☐ Other Concerns in the Mental Health Setting

The sources of risk in psychiatric facilities are increasing. Some that warrant close scrutiny and corrective measures include:

- *Elopement.* As long as there have been psychiatric institutions, there has been elopement—patient escape to the outside. These events have the potential to generate tremendous adverse publicity and to spur protest from the community as neighborhood residents fear for their families, justifiably or not. The facility can also be held accountable for the actions of an escaped patient, particularly a committed or criminal patient.

  Consequently, the facility must enact stringent security measures. Guards should be employed, and the facility or unit safety function should establish a healthy, cooperative relationship with the security force. Security personnel can act as a valuable resource, particularly when they are made aware of the special needs of psychiatric patients. The facility should be designed to be secure, and periodic inspections should regularly determine the continuing security of the building.

  Equally important, every attempt should be made to provide as pleasant and unrestricted an atmosphere as possible for the patients. Patients should be provided with ample recreation, outdoor and indoor, that is consistent with treatment goals. Visits with family and friends should be allowed and, where possible, excursions should be available. Staff members should document and respond to frequently occurring patient complaints, and, above all, patients should always be treated with dignity and respect. Elopement is at least partially preventable through attention to patient comfort and concerns.
- *Credentialing.* Expanding regulatory control and publicity have centered on the professional ability of psychiatric staff to dispense high-quality

care. One problem in ensuring the competence of mental health facility staff is the numbers of different types of professionals providing care. Psychiatric care can involve such diverse professionals as physicians, nurses, psychologists, social workers, therapists, technicians, chaplains, volunteers, student interns, orderlies, and aides.

Many treatment methods—group therapy, for example—can be carried out by individuals with varying levels of education, training, and experience. It is important to note, however, that this diversity of personnel is desirable and, in some instances, required. For example, the Joint Commission requires psychiatric and long-term care facilities to provide related social work services as an adjunct to good care.

Many of the highly publicized cases of malpractice originate in charges that staff members were incompetent or should not have been privileged for a certain procedure. Predetermined criteria should establish the specific responsibilities and tasks for which privileges will be granted. Privileges should not be granted to a profession as a whole. Licensing varies from state to state, so those responsible should ascertain whether the individual is licensed to practice in their state. Finally, background checks are becoming increasingly necessary to discover previous charges of abuse or incompetence.

- *Training and education.* Because many identified problems in psychiatric care stem from or are exacerbated by inadequate employee training, training and education should be a priority for the mental health facility. The emphasis should be on increasing staff awareness, both of the unique traits of the patient population and of their own responses to patient behavior. In addition to traditional safety topics, employees should receive training in physical management, dealing with anger and stress, the proper use of controversial treatment methods, determining dangerousness in patients, suicide precautions, and other identified risk areas. The continuing education of professionals through advanced degrees, conferences, and seminars should be required and encouraged.
- *The need for teamwork.* A long-used treatment method in psychiatric care, the treatment team approach, has become more and more important in maintaining safety and reducing risks. In this traditional method, several professionals—nurses, physicians, therapists, social workers, and others—form a treatment team that works together and regularly meets to discuss patient progress and treatment options. Although this has always been an effective method, it has now also become a means of protecting the facility from liability and safety hazards. The members of the team can provide different perspectives, support or argue against the idea of one person (one person's opinion may be difficult to defend if the need should arise), and detect hazards another individual may not detect.
- *Diagnostic and assessment practices.* Because of the changeable and sometimes elusive nature of mental illness, diagnosis is often troublesome. Furthermore, patients' conditions can often change suddenly and dramatically, or sometimes imperceptibly. Staff must identify and keep up with the progress of patients in order to target treatment. For this reason, rigorous diagnostic and reassessment procedures should be in place. Crucial factors to consider include progress that may alter the desirability of restrictions, medications, transfer or discharge, and controversial treatment modalities. In addition, staff should carefully avoid "labeling" patients so that the diagnosis does not become a self-fulfilling prophecy. Figure 11-2 (see p. 159) provides a checklist for the ongoing monitoring and evaluation of care and treatment.

☐ Safety Inspection Guidelines

The mental health facility must also prevent accidents through basic safety measures. Local and state agencies have started to clamp down on psychiatric facilities with more stringent safety regulations and inspections. Therefore, mental health facilities should conduct regular inspections to ensure their compliance with applicable requirements. Some suggested inspection sites are described in the following sections. Standards may differ in each location, so individual facilities should check with regional agencies when planning an inspection.

General Psychiatric Facility

The following precautions apply to general psychiatric facilities:

- All exit doors should be alarmed.
- All fire pull boxes should be alarmed or tamper-resistant.
- All fire extinguishers should be in recessed, tamper-resistant boxes. Avoid the use of fire hoses, if possible.
- Security doors should be alarmed.
- All chute doors should be designed to prevent accidental entrance or injury.
- Windows should be inoperable and made of safety glass that can withstand substantial force.
- Smoking should be restricted to supervised areas only.
- All screws (including those used on electrical faceplates) should be tamper-resistant, requiring a special tool for removal.
- Base coving should be avoided because it becomes a place to hide contraband.

Patient Rooms

Because of the constant potential for sudden violence and suicide attempts, care should be taken in designing and maintaining patient rooms. Some essential considerations include the following:

- Mirrors should not consist of glass. Instead, they should be composed of acrylic plastic or stainless steel and should be firmly mounted to a structural wall.
- Light fixtures should be recessed and secured with tamperproof screws.
- All shower rods, shower heads, towel racks, clothing racks, and any other items that could be used in a hanging should be of the breakaway type or not capable of supporting body weight. They should be tested to be sure they cannot support even the weight of an adolescent or child, if the facility treats those age groups. Soft, bendable material should be used for these items, such as polyvinyl chloride (PVC) piping.
- Shower heads should be recessed so that no cords or pipes are available for destructive use.
- Any loose structural elements such as shelving or ledges should be removed or tightly secured.
- Any flowerpots should be plastic.
- Only three-pronged ground-fault circuit interrupter (GFCI) safety outlets should be used.
- Plastic bags of any kind, including trashcan liners, should not be placed or allowed to be brought into the rooms.

- Any strings or rope (including drawstrings for drapery) should be removed from rooms.
- Patients' rooms should be checked regularly and thoroughly for dangerous items that patients may have hidden, including sharp objects, rope, and plastic bags.
- All furniture should be secured to the structure.
- Windows should not be open and should be made of safety glass. Bars on the outside may be needed.

Control or Holding Room

Most psychiatric facilities and units within general care hospitals have a safe room where aggressive or suicidal patients may be held. Even the most seemingly innocuous items in this room can pose a serious safety hazard, for patients may be desperate to hurt themselves or others. Consequently, these rooms should be designed to protect both the patient and others in the facility and community. In addition to the measures outlined in the previous section, the following additional precautions should be taken in designing or improving the security of the control or holding room:

- Only a molded foam rubber mattress and box spring should be used. The bed should have no other framing.
- The room should be windowless, if possible. If there is a window, it should be heavily protected.
- The room shape should include as few protruding corners as possible.
- The door should be made of bonded wood core or other approved material and should contain a wire glass window for monitoring the patient.
- In order to assist in monitoring, a closed-circuit television camera with a remote monitor may be installed. It should be recessed or positioned out of reach of the patient. If it is not recessed, a secured steel casing should surround the camera. An intercom should enable staff members to communicate with the patient.
- Thin inside walls in the room may allow the patient to break through a single-wall construction. Especially for walls of 1/2-inch or 5/8-inch thickness and of drywall construction, some additional protection may need to be provided, such as plywood strips with Sheetrock™ facing.
- Bathrooms inside the room should not be capable of being locked from the inside unless there is an emergency override on the outside and the door swings both ways.
- Air vents should be incapable of supporting body weight.
- The room should not have dropped ceilings.

□ Conclusion

Like other health care facilities, psychiatric institutions assume a responsibility for maintaining a safe and secure environment for their patients. Therefore, the other elements of safety described in this text should be adapted to the psychiatric facility's overall safety program. These elements include disaster preparedness, fire safety, hazardous materials safety, compliance with regulatory requirements, accident prevention, incident reporting, and patient safety. By implementing such a comprehensive safety and risk reduction program, the progressive mental health facility will ensure its ability to meet accelerating demands and to continue to serve the community well and profitably.

Figure 11-1. Patient Rights in Mental Health and Long-Term Care Facilities

Patients have basic rights that the facility has a responsibility to uphold. If the patient is not considered legally competent to understand or exercise them, these rights transfer to the guardian or other person designated to act on the patient's behalf. These are patients' rights to:

1. Be treated with consideration, respect, and full recognition of their dignity and individuality.
2. Receive information on their rights and responsibilities and any changes or amendments to these rights.
3. Be encouraged and assisted to exercise their rights.
4. Be provided with information on services available in the facility, the cost of these services, and the right to file complaints concerning charges they believe are unjustified.
5. Be given the opportunity to participate in the planning of their care and treatment.
6. Be offered the least controversial, restrictive, or invasive treatment method available and effective for the condition.
7. Refuse any treatment.
8. Manage their own personal finances.
9. Be suitably dressed at all times and be given assistance in maintaining good hygiene.
10. With their families, be informed of progress and changes in treatment plans.
11. Be free from abuse and unnecessary physical and chemical restraint.
12. Be protected during an emergency when they cannot protect themselves.
13. Receive privacy and confidentiality.
14. Be allowed freedom of communication and correspondence with and from others.
15. Participate in activities to the full extent of their abilities.

Figure 11-2. Checklist for Monitoring and Evaluating Care and Treatment

The following questions can be used in the monitoring of each of the steps in the treatment process:

Diagnosis

- Is the diagnosis justified by:
  - The patient's presenting/chief complaint?
  - The patient's symptoms as identified in the psychiatric assessment?
  - The patient's history of prior conditions/disorders?

Admission

- Is the need for patient admission justified by:
  - The patient's presenting/chief complaint?
  - The patient's symptoms as identified in the psychiatric assessment?
  - The patient's history?

Diagnostic assessments

- Are diagnostic assessments justified by the clinical information available?
  - Are special therapeutic assessments (occupational/physical therapy, speech and language, and so on) justified by the clinical information available?
  - Does the patient's clinical status indicate the need for diagnostic assessments that were not ordered/performed?
- Are laboratory, X-ray, and other ancillary diagnostic tests justified by the patient's physical examination/history?
  - Are these test results made available in a timely manner?
  - Are abnormal test results noted and addressed appropriately?
- Are psychiatric/medical consultations justified by the patient's clinical condition?
  - Are consultations completed promptly?
  - Are consultants' recommendations addressed?

Treatment plan

- Is the treatment plan justified by the patient's clinical condition?
  - Is it consistent with the diagnosis?
  - Does it support the need for treatment at this facility and/or at this program/departmental level?
  - Does it respond to the problems identified in the diagnostic assessments?
- Are short-term goals consistent with:
  - The patient's diagnosis?
  - The patient's strengths as determined in diagnostic assessments?
- Are long-term goals consistent with:
  - The patient's diagnosis?
  - The patient's strengths as determined in the diagnostic assessments?
  - The patient's progress?
- Are nursing care plans or other mental health professionals' care plans consistent with the overall treatment plan?

Treatments

- Are prescribed treatments appropriate in view of:
  - The patient's diagnosis?
  - The patient's clinical condition?
  - The treatment plan?
  - The treatment goals?
- Are prescribed medications appropriate in view of:
  - The patient's diagnosis?
  - The patient's clinical condition?
  - The treatment plan?
  - The treatment goals?
- Are prescribed treatments carried out:
  - By the proper individuals?
  - At the proper times?
  - In the proper manner?
  - In the least restrictive, most appropriate manner?
  - By the least intrusive method?

Continued on next page

Figure 11-2. (Continued)

Patient's response

- Do treatments have the desired effect or achieve the desired response from the patient?
- Is the treatment plan changed in keeping with changes in the patient's clinical condition?
  - Are changes in the treatment plan justified by the patient's response to treatment?
- Is the treatment plan changed in keeping with the patient's lack of response to treatment?

Discharge

- Is the discharge plan consistent with:
  - The treatment plan?
  - The patient's treatment progress?
  - The patient's need for social support after treatment as identified in the social worker's diagnostic assessment?
- Is the patient's status at discharge in keeping with treatment plan goals?

Aftercare

- Do aftercare plans:
  - Sufficiently prepare the patient for follow-up?
  - Sufficiently prepare the follow-up care facility for the patient?

Source: Reprinted, with permission, from Joseph, E. D. Strengthening risk management in psychiatric facilities. *Perspectives in Healthcare Risk Management* 8(4):16–17, Fall 1988.

Chapter 12

Program Integration and Evaluation

The measures described in the preceding chapters of this book are crucial to the development and implementation of a comprehensive safety program. However, to ensure the continued vitality and efficacy of the program—10 years, 1 year, or even 6 months later—the facility must institute a process of self-review through which the effects, benefits, problems, and new goals of the safety program are identified and reassessed. Because both society and the health care environment are changing rapidly, programs implemented today may not be appropriate to concerns emerging two years later *unless* there is a process of periodic review and evaluation.

A newly introduced safety program, even with the full support of management and administration, will not reach its full potential unless it is integrated into other services and departments and becomes a natural part of the facility's daily routine. Safety cannot be allowed to stand apart from the mission and day-to-day activities of the facility, nor can safety personnel be viewed as outsiders to normal procedures. Consequently, a major goal in implementing the safety program will be to integrate safety functions into all patient care procedures and to gain the full understanding and commitment of the staff. The importance of these processes to the continued success of the safety program cannot be overemphasized.

☐ Regular Inspections and Monitoring

Integration and evaluation of the safety program takes place through regular inspections and monitoring. The value of consistent assessment is reinforced by the Joint Commission on Accreditation of Healthcare Organizations. Most of the Commission's major standards include the requirement that actions be "evaluated for effectiveness," that problems be uncovered, and that solutions be implemented. Without this kind of follow-up, the safety officers and safety committee might remain unaware of various failings or outdated elements of the program, such as elements of the program that may be resented or viewed as a nuisance by personnel or a procedure that may be ineffective or outdated and need rethinking. Whatever the reason for less-than-effective safety measures, periodic inspections and ongoing monitoring can identify problems, which can then be resolved.

A thorough facilitywide evaluation, similar to the needs assessment described in chapter 1, should be undertaken six months after implementation of the comprehensive safety management program and annually thereafter. The chief coordinators of these reassessments are safety department personnel and the safety committee. The goals of the periodic evaluations are to determine whether procedures have been fully implemented, whether they are accomplishing what they set out to accomplish, and whether they are achieving this in an acceptable manner. This review should utilize the results of the original needs assessment as a basis for comparison—including the final needs assessment report and all of the records that were used. Documents from before and after the program's implementation that can be used include the following:

- Incident reports
- Safety committee minutes
- Voluntary and regulatory agency survey reports
- Insurance company inspection results
- Workers' compensation statistics
- New and old policies and procedures
- Data tracking results

Former and current records should be compared to discover progress or stalled implementation. For example, data tracking will show the incidence of various types of accidents, so the effects of new practices can be evaluated. The documents should be reviewed not only for their ability to demonstrate reduced accident rates, claims, and so forth but also for the purpose of organizing and keeping track of aggregate data showing broader trends.

In addition to reviewing these documents, safety personnel evaluating the program, including safety committee members, should also walk through the facility. The visual inspection, preferably unannounced, can uncover structural and equipment hazards as well as unsafe practices. Inspectors should talk with employees about their reactions to the practicality and effectiveness of various program elements. When employees are found to be using unsafe procedures, they should be asked for an honest explanation, rather than just being rebuked. Sometimes procedures are impractical or too time-consuming, or employees have not been adequately trained in using them. Employees are often reluctant to express these concerns unless asked in the context of helping to improve the program.

Department managers and supervisors can also monitor daily practices. When employees are not working safely, the managers should determine why in a nonthreatening manner. Managers should assure employees that if the problem is one of poorly designed policies and procedures or insufficient training, there will be no reprisals. The managers and supervisors can explain that employee input is valuable to the sustained success of the safety program. This communication is essential, for line employees are the ones most responsible for the daily implementation of the program. Another way to assess employee reactions to procedures is in training. Questions on in-service evaluation forms can ask what employees think of the measures and the luck they are having using them.

Even though the first evaluation should take place approximately six months after the program's implementation, dramatic results should not be expected too soon. Just developing and implementing the policies and procedures, introducing them to staff, and training employees in carrying them out may require a year or more. It may take some time just to catch up with liabilities that existed prior to the introduction of the program. The concrete economic dividends can often be slow to materialize at first, partly because insurance carriers may wait to reduce premiums until the safety management program displays significant statistical results. The point is that comprehensive safety management is a long-term process requiring perseverance and, to some degree, vision. Up-front costs (financial and otherwise) may seem burdensome, but the long-term rewards will outweigh any earlier sacrifices.

Without the tools of evaluation and consistent monitoring, the program could suffer after the initial excitement of its inauguration. Thorough review and measurement of results revitalizes the process and answers questions about what the program has accomplished and where future effort should be focused.

□ Obstacles to Implementation

The most common obstacles to the successful implementation of a safety program result from a lack of enthusiasm and teamwork, dwindling availability of funds, and changes within the facility.

Lack of Enthusiasm and Teamwork

Lack of enthusiasm, commitment, and teamwork among employees can be the fatal blow to a faltering program. However, this lack of involvement can be overcome through continued efforts at communication with and motivation of employees—from the program's introduction through its annual evaluation.

The seeds for permanent commitment to the program should be sown in the initial stages of development. If administrators, managers, and supervisors have properly performed each of the steps in the program's development and implementation, employees will, at this stage, have already accepted the program, at least in principle. Crucial steps that should not have been overlooked include:

- Obtaining publicized administration support
- Encouraging employee participation in planning processes
- Encouraging employee involvement in safety committee actions
- Considering safety-consciousness in hiring
- Including discussions of safety in orientation
- Providing ongoing safety training for the different levels of staff
- Stressing continued interaction about the program between employees and supervisors

If carefully executed, these early steps will provide a firm foundation on which to build good safety practices.

At this stage, employees may accept the existence of the program—at least as a bulk of administration policies and procedures—but they may remain skeptical as to whether the philosophy and new procedures should really be part of their jobs. They may wonder whether the program is not just a passing fad. Consequently, it is crucial at this time to emphasize that the program still has unwavering support from top administration. Another statement signed by the chief executive officer (CEO) (as a follow-up to the original statement of support discussed in chapter 1) could outline the ongoing efforts in safety and reiterate moral and financial support. Department managers and supervisors are responsible for seeing to it that safety really does become a component of every job description and a determinant of the quality of employee performance. Helping employees see that their performance is judged in this context becomes an effective motivator.

Employees should know that their efforts are not in vain. Incident reports and employee suggestions or complaints should receive prompt follow-up. Management should serve as an example of sound safety habits, so that an implicit double standard does not become a source of staff resentment. The safety committee should regularly review all information on hazards and eliminate them.

Another effective way of building teamwork and commitment is through incentive programs. Workers who consistently observe prudent safety practices and employees who customarily display a spirit of teamwork and cooperation should be rewarded. The criteria for awards can vary, and facilities should experiment with what works best for them. Some actions that may warrant recognition include having no lost work time injuries over a certain period of time, performing a safe action in the face of an emergency or serious risk, having perfect attendance at safety training in-services, or providing usable suggestions for program improvement.

The type of incentive provided might differ depending on staff characteristics and previous experience. Praise from supervisors, managers, and administrators can be a powerful incentive in itself. Another almost fail-safe motivator (if used correctly) is a pay incentive for no lost work time injuries. Using monetary incentives can avoid the problem of discrepancies over what constitutes a good prize. In addition, many organizations and companies offer cost-effective and creative incentive packages that facilities can buy and use.

An additional reinforcement (discussed in detail in chapter 10) is training. Regular safety training keeps safety on the mind, introduces new skills, and encourages the enhancement of rusty ones. Repeated training should go hand in hand with evaluation in ensuring that safety becomes integrated into the overall management system and work ethic of the facility.

Various other reinforcements exist, most of which derive from the idea that providing visual reminders can cause employees to remember safety or stop and think before acting in an unsafe manner. Among the most widely used reinforcements are posters. Timely posters that do not treat employees as children and that employ humor and sophistication can be quite effective. They attract attention while conveying a message. They should be positioned in a high-traffic area and be near the hazard to which they refer. Posters should be regularly replaced to prevent them from fading into the scenery. Other visual reminders—which can also serve as rewards or incentives—include pins, hats, pens, and T-shirts with safety messages. The thoughtful use of rewards, visual reminders, praise, incentives, and routine interaction with employees can go a long way toward engendering the commitment and teamwork essential to program success.

It is natural for the enthusiasm of everyone involved in the program to falter somewhat as the program becomes familiar and routine. For this reason, the constant commitment of employees should never be taken for granted. There should be a set of built-in motivational checkpoints to boost flagging interest. In evaluating the program and removing hindrances to implementation, the focus will always be on the people in the organization. Safety management is a human process best approached through and with the cooperation of the facility's diverse personnel.

Dwindling Funds

A factor that frequently impedes the progress of safety is dwindling funds. The safety management program may become the first target of budget cuts, for its start-up costs may seem considerable in relation to its immediate economic benefits. This logic is shortsighted and can jeopardize the facility in the long run. Before reducing funds, the CEO, the administrators, and others involved should look at their reasons for initiating a safety effort and identify the consequences that will result from reduced funding. The bottom-line reason for safety is twofold: humanitarian and financial. Without the program, liabilities and losses resulting from unsafe conditions will continue to rise in proportion to escalating risks, defeating the purpose of saving money by cutting funding.

If cuts in the safety program are unavoidable or if across-the-board reductions are necessary, the safety committee should meet to decide which program elements can most survive a cut, based on the priorities identified in the original assessment and most of all, in the recent evaluation. For example, if the facility had been cited for improper hazardous waste handling procedures, the hazardous materials management program should be shielded from reductions in funding. As the safety management program begins to show more quantifiable results, cuts should become less justifiable.

Changes within the Facility

Modifications in services or other processes can make some policies and procedures obsolete and can necessitate new ones. For example, as the demographics of society change, facilities may move toward expanded services for the elderly, whose needs differ from those of younger patients. Equipment relying on advanced technology will become increasingly commonplace, requiring stepped-up training for users and stricter preventive maintenance. Regulations and other requirements are modified almost daily, calling for alterations in practices that were once routine.

The safety management program should be designed to adapt to such changes—both sudden and gradual. This can be accomplished through continued program evaluation, as outlined in this chapter.

□ Conclusion

Establishing a system whereby the value and effectiveness of the safety management program is periodically and comprehensively reassessed provides the key to the lasting success of the program. Evaluation depends on honest self-review by everyone involved, requiring each employee of the facility to appraise frankly his or her own role and ability to fulfill that function. It is a time for the organization as a whole to congratulate itself and for the institution's leaders to praise and reward their staff for forbearance and cooperation. It is also a time to peer into the future and plan for new challenges. Drawing on a sound safety management program that is capable of regular self-evaluation and change, the facility and its staff can face the future with confidence and pride.

Appendix A
List of Organizations

Agency for Toxic Substances and Disease Registry
1600 Clifton Road, N.E.
Atlanta, GA 30333
404/454-4630

American Association of Homes for the Aging
1050 17th Street, N.W., Suite 770
Washington, DC 20036
202/296-5960

American Health Care Association
1200 15th Street, N.W.
Washington, DC 20005
202/842-4444

American Hospital Association
840 North Lake Shore Drive
Chicago, IL 60611
312/280-6000

American National Standards Institute
1430 Broadway
New York, NY 10018
212/354-3300

American Society of Safety Engineers
850 Busse Highway
Park Ridge, IL 60068
312/692-4121

American Society for Training and Development
600 Maryland Avenue, S.W., Suite 305
Washington, DC 20024
202/362-1498

Centers for Disease Control
1600 Clifton Road, N.E.
Atlanta, GA 30333
404/639-3311

Compressed Gas Association, Inc.
1235 Jefferson Davis Highway
Arlington, VA 22202
703/979-0900

Department of Transportation
Materials Transportation Bureau
Information Services Division
Washington, DC 20590
202/366-4488

Federal Emergency Management Agency
P.O. Box 70274
Washington, DC 20472
202/646-2500

Federal Register
Superintendent of Documents
U.S. Government Printing Office
Washington, DC 20402
202/783-3238

Joint Commission on Accreditation of Healthcare Organizations
875 N. Michigan Avenue
Chicago, IL 60611
312/642-6061

National Fire Protection Association
Batterymarch Park
Quincy, MA 02269
800/544-3555

National Restaurant Association
311 First Street, N.W.
Washington, DC 20001
202/331-5900

National Safety Council
444 N. Michigan Avenue
Chicago, IL 60611
312/527-4800

Occupational Safety and Health Administration
U.S. Department of Labor
Washington, DC 20402
202/523-8063

Practicioner Reporting System
United States Pharmacopoeia
12601 Twinbrook Parkway
Rockville, MD 20852
800/638-6725

Underwriters Laboratories
333 Pfingsten Road
Northbrook, IL 60062
312/272-8800

U.S. Environmental Protection Agency
Office of Solid Waste and Emergency Response
Washington, DC 20460
202/382-4700

U.S. Food and Drug Administration
5600 Fishers Lane
Rockville, MD 20857
301/443-1544

U.S. Nuclear Regulatory Commission
1717 H Street
Washington, DC 20555
301/492-7000

Appendix B

Glossary of Abbreviations

AHA American Hospital Association

AIDS Acquired Immunodeficiency Syndrome

CAA Clean Air Act of 1970

CDC Centers for Disease Control

CEPP Chemical Emergency Preparedness Program (EPA)

CERCLA Comprehensive Environmental Response Compensation Liability Act

CFR Code of Federal Regulations

CSHO Compliance Safety and Health Officer

CWA Clean Water Act of 1977

DOL Department of Labor

DOT Department of Transportation

ECT Electroconvulsive Therapy

EMS Emergency Medical Services

EPA U.S. Environmental Protection Agency

FAA Federal Aviation Authority

HBV Hepatitis B Virus

HHS Department of Health and Human Services

HIV Human Immunodeficiency Virus

JCAHO Joint Commission on Accreditation of Healthcare Organizations (Joint Commission)

LASER Light Amplification by Stimulated Emission of Radiation

MSDS Material Safety Data Sheet

NFPA National Fire Protection Association

NIOSH National Institute for Occupational Safety and Health

NSC National Safety Council

NTP National Toxicology Program

OES Office of Emergency Services

OSHA Occupational Safety and Health Administration

PPE Personal Protective Equipment

RCRA Resource Conservation and Recovery Act

RQ Reportable Quantity

SARA Superfund Amendments and Reauthorization Act of 1986

SIC Standard Industrial Code

TPQ Threshold Planning Quantity

TSCA Toxic Substances Control Act of 1976

Appendix C
Safety Inspection Checklist

Item	Yes	No	Comments on Deficiencies Noted and Action Required	Date Corrected
General Safety Suggestions Is there a safety management program designed to provide a physical environment free of hazards and to manage staff activities to reduce the risk of injury?				
Is there a life safety program designed to protect patients, employees, visitors, and property from fire and other disasters?				
Does the program provide for the safe use of buildings and grounds?				
Is the facility in compliance with the appropriate edition of the Life Safety Code of the National Fire Protection Association (NFPA)?				
Is lighting sufficient?				
Are shades clean?				
Are surplus lights removed?				
Is ventilation satisfactory?				

Source: Adapted, with permission, from National Safety Council. *Long Term Care Safety Management Manual: A Handbook for Practical Application.* Chicago: National Safety Council, 1987, pp. 135–65.

Item	Yes	No	Comments on Deficiencies Noted and Action Required	Date Corrected
Is the building (floors, windows, and doors) kept in good repair?				
Is paint in rooms, on machines, and on equipment in good condition?				
Are routine inspections of equipment scheduled for proper maintenance?				
Are equipment, materials, or supplies removed when they are not used or become obsolete?				
Are unused materials, wiring, piping, fittings, electrical fixtures, motors, etc., stored properly?				
Is storage properly arranged: For materials?				
For working space?				
For grouping similar things together?				
For prevention of water loss?				
For ease of access?				
Are cabinets provided for small tools, buckets, brooms, brushes, shovels, mops, etc.?				
Is floor storage discouraged?				
Is storage on ledges, in corners, tops of cabinets, tops of lockers, radiators, etc., eliminated?				
Is the department provided with fire extinguishers?				
Are fire doors, aisles, and exits kept clear?				
Is hazardous equipment properly guarded?				
Are warning signs posted?				
Are employees observing "No Smoking" restrictions?				

Source: Adapted, with permission, from National Safety Council. *Long Term Care Safety Management Manual: A Handbook for Practical Application.* Chicago: National Safety Council, 1987, pp. 135–65.

Item	**Yes**	**No**	**Comments on Deficiencies Noted and Action Required**	**Date Corrected**
Have all employees been provided information to protect them from the effects of working with hazardous chemicals (OSHA Hazard Communication Standard—Right-to-Know)?				
Are Material Safety Data Sheets (MSDSs) readily available?				
Has a program been designed to safely manage hazardous/infectious wastes?				
Is all storage at least 18 inches below sprinkler heads so that sprinkler system will work properly in the event of a fire?				
Housekeeping Department Are electric cords and plugs, lamps, and heating pads in good condition?				
Are overhead lighting units in good condition?				
Are floors washed or waxed during quiet periods rather than during rush hours?				
Are dry areas or aisles left for persons to walk on by cleaning one side at a time?				
Are wet areas blocked off and is a sign posted to warn persons approaching?				
Are floors rinsed and dried thoroughly after cleaning?				
Are nonskid waxes or polishes used?				
If lightweight rugs or throw rugs are used, do they have rubber backing?				
Is broken glass immediately removed from floors? Same for flower petals, gum, candy, and cigarette wrappers?				
Are the tops of stepladders, cabinets, or lockers empty and free of articles?				

Source: Adapted, with permission, from National Safety Council. *Long Term Care Safety Management Manual: A Handbook for Practical Application.* Chicago: National Safety Council, 1987, pp. 135–65.

Item	Yes	No	Comments on Deficiencies Noted and Action Required	Date Corrected
Are all stepladders in safe condition?				
Do portable ladders have safety feet?				
Are wastebaskets held by the sides and emptied over a refuse bag?				
Are the proper tools used for opening containers?				
Are protruding nails, metal strapping, and wires removed from all boxes, barrels, and crates before handling?				
Are oils, waxes, sweeping compounds, and all flammable supplies and materials properly stored?				
Are proper provisions made for taking care of water on the floor of the dishwashing room?				
Are link mats or other types of corrugated rubber matting used?				
Are employees properly instructed as to the course of action in case of fire or other emergency?				
Are employees properly instructed regarding any hazards in the work required of them?				
Are there plastic liners in all garbage pails?				
Are all garbage pails covered?				
Are liquids disposed of only in sinks or, where appropriate, in safety cans?				
Are sharp objects never put in garbage pails?				
Are there special boxes for disposal of needles and sharps?				
Is the trash can in a patient's room used only for paper waste?				

Source: Adapted, with permission, from National Safety Council. *Long Term Care Safety Management Manual: A Handbook for Practical Application.* Chicago: National Safety Council, 1987, pp. 135–65.

Item	Yes	No	Comments on Deficiencies Noted and Action Required	Date Corrected
Are employees instructed never to stand on the top two steps of a ladder?				
Is any equipment or furniture that is heavy or awkward to handle lifted or moved by more than one person or by mechanical devices?				
Do all electrical appliances such as vacuums and polishers have grounded connections?				
When floors are being scrubbed or polished, is the area identified as being slippery by posting or roping off the area?				
Is all trash handled as if hazardous items were contained in the refuse?				
Are all cleaning solutions clearly labeled with ingredients and warnings indicated?				
Does the housekeeping director inspect the institution regularly?				
Are mops available in all departments for emergency drying of leakage, spillage, etc.?				
Are dustpans available?				
Are drinking fountains, showers, baths, and lavatories cleaned daily?				
Laundry Department Are bleaches or other strong solutions handled and stored safely?				
Do those who handle such solutions take proper precautions to protect eyes and hands?				
Are steam lines insulated to prevent burns?				
Is the safety on the feed roll of the flat ironer in good working order?				

Source: Adapted, with permission, from National Safety Council. *Long Term Care Safety Management Manual: A Handbook for Practical Application.* Chicago: National Safety Council, 1987, pp. 135–65.

Item	Yes	No	Comments on Deficiencies Noted and Action Required	Date Corrected
Are extractors inspected regularly for safe working conditions?				
Are hot-water temperatures limited to 180° F?				
Is contagious linen properly handled in safe bags with special markers?				
Are employees who sort contagious linen properly protected with gowns, masks, and gloves?				
Is clean linen handled differently from soiled linen to prevent contamination?				
Are floors kept clear of standing water, grease, lint, etc.?				
Is lint removed regularly and frequently from dryers?				
Is excess oil and grease removed regularly on machines and equipment to prevent accumulation?				
Are nonskid mats or flooring provided in wet areas?				
Do employees wear nonskid shoes?				
Is there a facility procedure for preventing sharp objects from being left in laundry?				
Is all laundry handled as if hazardous instruments were present in the laundry?				
Are portable air fans adequately guarded and properly grounded?				
Is hot equipment shielded so employees are protected from the heat?				
Do employees have easy access to water and cool air to combat heat stress?				

Source: Adapted, with permission, from National Safety Council. *Long Term Care Safety Management Manual: A Handbook for Practical Application.* Chicago: National Safety Council, 1987, pp. 135–65.

From *Safety Guide for Healthcare Institutions*, 4th edition, published by American Hospital Publishing, copyright 1989.

Item	Yes	No	Comments on Deficiencies Noted and Action Required	Date Corrected
Is there a required cleanup procedure and disinfectant soap available in the laundry?				
Is dirty laundry picked up and sorted daily?				
Are carts used only for dirty laundry, or clean laundry, never for both?				
Are linen transport carts labeled "soiled" and "clean"?				
Are these carts cleaned with a germicide on a regular basis?				
Is the clean linen room kept dusted, vacuumed, and clean?				
Are emergency instructions posted?				
Is the laundry room provided with adequate fire extinguishers?				
Is adequate aisle space maintained?				
Are instructions for the proper operation of laundry equipment posted?				
Is equipment so placed as to permit safe egress from all areas of the room?				
Maintenance Department Are all ladders in safe condition?				
Are portable ladders unpainted and equipped with safety feet?				
Are all hand tools returned to their proper places after use and in good condition?				
Are wrench jaws in good condition so that they will not slip?				
Are wrenches available in various sizes so that the proper size is available for each job?				

Source: Adapted, with permission, from National Safety Council. *Long Term Care Safety Management Manual: A Handbook for Practical Application.* Chicago: National Safety Council, 1987, pp. 135–65.

Item	Yes	No	Comments on Deficiencies Noted and Action Required	Date Corrected
Are chisels, punches, and pins removed when their heads are mushroomed, making them unsafe to use?				
Are hammers removed when their heads are chipped or when handles are loose or cracked?				
Are tools always kept out of reach of patients?				
Are tools used only by qualified personnel?				
Are tools in good, safe working order?				
Aisles Are aisles clear, uncluttered, and well lighted?				
Is nonskid wax used?				
Stairways Are stairways kept free and unobstructed?				
Are treads in good order with nonskid nosings?				
Is riser height and tread width uniform?				
Are stairways, corridors, and ramps equipped with required handrails?				
General Are maintenance employees properly instructed as to course of action in case of fire or other emergency?				
Do they all know the location of fire extinguishers?				
Do they know what type of extinguisher to use for different types of fires?				
Are all exit signs illuminated?				

Source: Adapted, with permission, from National Safety Council. *Long Term Care Safety Management Manual: A Handbook for Practical Application.* Chicago: National Safety Council, 1987, pp. 135–65.

From *Safety Guide for Healthcare Institutions*, 4th edition, published by American Hospital Publishing, copyright 1989.

Item	Yes	No	Comments on Deficiencies Noted and Action Required	Date Corrected
Do all exit doors swing outward?				
Do exit doors have "crash hardware"?				
Do they unlock from the inside?				
Is the entire exit area inspected periodically for safety hazards?				
Is water set at a safe temperature in patient care areas?				
Yard Are drives clear and pavement in good condition?				
Are walks in good repair and unobstructed?				
Are direction signs: Properly lighted?				
Properly placed?				
Easily read?				
In good condition?				
Are precautions taken to prevent icicles, snow, etc., from falling on people below?				
Are guardrails and gratings arranged to prevent falling into areaways and stairwells?				
Are they in good repair?				
General Are materials stacked neatly and not scattered in aisles and over floors?				
Are there blade guards on table saws, band saws, and radial arm saws?				
Are metal ladders never used by employees working on electrical equipment or wiring or changing light bulbs?				
Are broken ladders destroyed, or tagged and removed from service until repaired?				

Source: Adapted, with permission, from National Safety Council. *Long Term Care Safety Management Manual: A Handbook for Practical Application.* Chicago: National Safety Council, 1987, pp. 135–65.

Item	**Yes**	**No**	**Comments on Deficiencies Noted and Action Required**	**Date Corrected**
Are battery-charging areas designated "No Smoking" and well ventilated?				
Is gasoline-powered equipment operated in well-ventilated areas?				
Are protective clothing and equipment provided for and worn by all employees exposed to hazards requiring protection, such as: Gloves—for handling hot, wet, or sharp objects and chemicals?				
Eye and face protection—for protection from chips, sparks, glass, and splashes?				
Hearing protection—for protection from noise sources?				
Local exhaust ventilation— for wood dust (to remove fine dust when sanding)?				
Are oxygen cylinders in storage separated from fuel-gas cylinders and combustible materials, especially oil or grease?				
Are full and empty cylinders stored separately?				
Are all compressed gas cylinders chained or secured safely?				
Are oxygen and fuel gases separated by at least 20 feet?				
Are all cylinders stored away from heat sources such as radiators, steam pipes, and direct sunlight?				
Are all cylinders kept free of grease?				
Are trash compactors operable only in the closed position?				

Source: Adapted, with permission, from National Safety Council. *Long Term Care Safety Management Manual: A Handbook for Practical Application.* Chicago: National Safety Council, 1987, pp. 135–65.

Item	Yes	No	Comments on Deficiencies Noted and Action Required	Date Corrected
Are there safety measures or devices on trash compactors (such as two-hand controls, electric eyes, or emergency shut-off bars) to minimize risk of injury?				
Is personal protective equipment worn when insulation is being replaced to avoid inhalation of asbestos and glass fibers?				
Is there adequate ventilation in areas being painted?				
Do emergency repairs take precedence over routine work?				
Has an equipment management program been developed?				
Does the equipment management program assess and control the risks of fixed and portable equipment used for diagnosis, treatment, and monitoring of patients?				
Is there a utilities management program designed to assure the operational reliability and respond to failures of utility systems that support the patient care environment?				
Does it include: Systems for electrical distributors?				
Emergency power?				
Vertical and horizontal transport?				
Heating?				
Ventilating and air-conditioning?				
Plumbing?				
Boiler and steam?				
Medical gas?				
Medical/surgical vacuum?				

Source: Adapted, with permission, from National Safety Council. *Long Term Care Safety Management Manual: A Handbook for Practical Application*. Chicago: National Safety Council, 1987, pp. 135–65.

Item	Yes	No	Comments on Deficiencies Noted and Action Required	Date Corrected
Nursing Department Are provisions made for safe disposal of broken syringes, needles, and empty bottles wherever medications and treatments are prepared or given?				
If employees have to use any type of stepladder to reach storage shelves, are these ladders or stools nontipping, skidproof, and capable of bearing weight?				
Is storage space provided for ladders and stools when not in use?				
Are employees instructed how to properly lift patients?				
Are extension cords used anywhere?				
If so, could they be eliminated by better and more adequate wiring?				
Are electrical cords in good condition and without worn places?				
Are all rooms where medications are prepared properly lighted to prevent errors due to poor visibility?				
Are floors free from breaks, loose tiles or linoleum, or any obstruction that might cause people to stumble or fall?				
Is plumbing in good repair, preventing water seepage or condensation that could cause a wet or slippery floor?				
Are handles provided on all mattresses?				
Are there doors or locks on all medicine cabinets?				
Are medical gas cylinders chained to the carrier to prevent tipping? Are they chained to prevent tipping while in storage?				

Source: Adapted, with permission, from National Safety Council. *Long Term Care Safety Management Manual: A Handbook for Practical Application.* Chicago: National Safety Council, 1987, pp. 135–65.

From *Safety Guide for Healthcare Institutions*, 4th edition, published by American Hospital Publishing, copyright 1989.

Item	Yes	No	Comments on Deficiencies Noted and Action Required	Date Corrected
Are tanks secured even when empty?				
Is a valve protection cap in place when oxygen cylinder is not in use?				
Are "No Smoking" signs posted on oxygen tents when in use?				
Are fire extinguishers available at strategic places?				
Do employees know the location of the nearest fire pull alarm box?				
Are extinguishers inspected regularly?				
Are employees aware of the location of the extinguisher nearest them?				
Do they know how to use it?				
Are employees fully instructed in the proper manner of lifting, handling, and carrying?				
Are they evaluated based on proper follow-through?				
Are passageways and halls free of boxes or other articles being stored?				
Are floors treated with nonslip material and is this treatment maintained?				
Are electrical cords for lights, TVs, radios, and patient monitoring equipment placed so as to prevent tripping hazards?				
Are needles and other sharp instruments discarded only in designated containers?				
Are microwave ovens cleaned regularly?				
Are acids and other chemicals properly labeled and safely stored and handled?				

Source: Adapted, with permission, from National Safety Council. *Long Term Care Safety Management Manual: A Handbook for Practical Application.* Chicago: National Safety Council, 1987, pp. 135–65.

Item	Yes	No	Comments on Deficiencies Noted and Action Required	Date Corrected
Are spills (water, flowers, food, etc.) cleaned up promptly?				
Physical Therapy Department Is all equipment used in the department regularly checked to prevent electrical shock and to prevent burns due to faulty thermostats or regulators?				
If nonprofessional employees are working in this department, are they aware of the dangers inherent in some of this equipment?				
Are floors tested for nonslipping qualities where instructions are given for walking with crutches, canes, and various types of walkers?				
Are provisions made for testing water, oil, or paraffin temperatures?				
Are mops available to clean up water on the floor where baths are given?				
Are ropes, pulleys, straps, etc., in good condition?				
Are all brackets attached to wall or ceiling firmly fixed?				
Storerooms Are storerooms well lighted?				
Are storerooms orderly?				
Are exits and aisles of storerooms clear at all times?				
Are rubbish, empty cartons, and paper disposed of immediately?				
Are heavy items always stored on the lower shelves?				
Are spillage items always stored below eye level?				
Are objects that might roll blocked?				

Source: Adapted, with permission, from National Safety Council. *Long Term Care Safety Management Manual: A Handbook for Practical Application.* Chicago: National Safety Council, 1987, pp. 135–65.

Item	Yes	No	Comments on Deficiencies Noted and Action Required	Date Corrected
Are materials stored clear of sprinkler heads (at least 18 inches) and other fire-fighting equipment?				
When cases are stacked head high or higher, are the cases crisscrossed to eliminate danger of falling cases?				
Are flammable liquids: Stored in approved containers?				
Stored in safe quantities?				
Stored in approved cabinets?				
Are storage shelves adequate for the weight involved?				
Are stepladders, rather than "makeshifts," always used to stand on?				
Are all stepladders in safe condition?				
Do portable ladders have safety feet?				
Are employees lifting heavy objects in the proper way?				
Are corrugated cartons opened with a sharp knife or special cutting tool, rather than pried loose with the hand or fingers?				
Are fire extinguishers located in a conspicuous place?				
Are employees made aware of these extinguishers, and do they know how to use them?				
Is storage properly arranged with consideration for the following: Space for materials?				
Space for working?				
Similar things together?				
Prevention of water loss?				
Ease of access?				

Source: Adapted, with permission, from National Safety Council. *Long Term Care Safety Management Manual: A Handbook for Practical Application.* Chicago: National Safety Council, 1987, pp. 135–65.

Item	Yes	No	Comments on Deficiencies Noted and Action Required	Date Corrected
Is storage on ledges, in corners, on tops of cabinets, on tops of lockers, etc., eliminated?				
Are "No Smoking" rules enforced?				
All Food Service Areas *Walking Surfaces (floors, ramps, stairs)* Are all walking surfaces maintained in safe condition: Are walking surfaces free of broken or missing tiles, defective boards, and damaged cement?				
Are they covered or treated with skid-resistant and cleanable materials?				
Are they thoroughly mopped on a regular schedule (food preparation, serving, and dining areas at least three times a week; storage, receiving, and waste areas at least once a week)?				
Are spillage and breakage cleaned up immediately as seen?				
Is a routine inspection for these hazards made after each meal?				
Are aisles, corridors, exits, and stairs kept clear at all times?				
Equipment, Utensils, and Clothing—General Is there a monthly inspection for faulty or damaged equipment, utensils, and counter, wall, floor, and ceiling surfaces?				
Is there an established procedure for immediate employee reporting of faulty or damaged equipment, utensils, and counter surfaces?				
Is faulty or damaged equipment immediately removed from use?				

Source: Adapted, with permission, from National Safety Council. *Long Term Care Safety Management Manual: A Handbook for Practical Application.* Chicago: National Safety Council, 1987, pp. 135–65.

From *Safety Guide for Healthcare Institutions*, 4th edition, published by American Hospital Publishing, copyright 1989.

Item	Yes	No	Comments on Deficiencies Noted and Action Required	Date Corrected
Are employees forbidden to use equipment unless specifically trained in its use?				
Are there restrictions or guidelines on loose-fitting clothing, jewelry, or long hair to prevent entanglement in machinery, food contamination, or fire while near the range burners?				
Are all employees wearing sturdy, closed-toe, low-heeled shoes that minimize slips, falls, burns, and cuts?				
Are meat saws, slicers, and grinders properly assembled and guarded?				
Are tamps or push sticks used to feed food grinders and choppers?				
Are all needed items of protective clothing and equipment supplied to employees, and is their utilization required?				
Electrical Equipment— General Is all electrical equipment safely located, maintained, and operated: Is electrical equipment grounded either through a built-in three-wire system or by attachment of a separate ground wire?				
Is it double insulated?				
Is it inspected regularly by an electrician?				
Are switches recessed or otherwise guarded so that equipment cannot be started by someone accidentally leaning or brushing against the switch?				
Are switches located so that employees do not have to lean on or against metal equipment to reach them?				
Are switches located to enable rapid emergency cutoff?				

Source: Adapted, with permission, from National Safety Council. *Long Term Care Safety Management Manual: A Handbook for Practical Application.* Chicago: National Safety Council, 1987, pp. 135–65.

Item	Yes	No	Comments on Deficiencies Noted and Action Required	Date Corrected
Are guards provided to prevent injury from electric shock, rotating blades, etc.?				
Glass, China—General Are facilities and handling procedures for glass and china designed to minimize breakage: Are storage facilities convenient to washing, serving, and dining areas?				
Are storage facilities sufficient to provide shelf or rack space for the total supply (no "temporary" storage on counter or table surfaces)?				
Is china stored in short stacks?				
Are glassware and cups stored rim edge down?				
Are employees given the following safety instructions: Carry only small amounts at one time; use racks, carts, or both.				
Discard chipped or cracked glass and china immediately.				
Do not pick up broken pieces of glassware with the bare hands; sweep them up into a dustpan with a brush or dampened paper.				
Always drain the sink or pan before removing broken glass.				
Place broken glass and china in a marked receptacle that can be dumped—not one from which it must be handpicked.				
Remove tops from glass bottles before discarding them (to minimize the danger of glass exploding if it is accidentally burned).				
Do not stack glass tumblers one inside another.				

Source: Adapted, with permission, from National Safety Council. *Long Term Care Safety Management Manual: A Handbook for Practical Application.* Chicago: National Safety Council, 1987, pp. 135–65.

Item	Yes	No	Comments on Deficiencies Noted and Action Required	Date Corrected
Do not put silver in glass tumblers or pitchers.				
Do not chip ice in glass water pitchers.				
Do not place glassware on same racks or trays as silver and china.				
Do not use glassware for storage of tacks, pins, insecticides, and cleaning and washing powders or solutions.				
Receiving, Waste Disposal, and Storage Areas—General Is each employee instructed in correct methods of lifting and handling for various types of containers?				
Is adequate equipment for handling bulk supplies provided: For opening crates, barrels, cartons (hammer, wire cutter, pliers, and cardboard carton openers)?				
For moving bulk supplies (hand trucks, dollies)?				
Is protective equipment provided for employees and its use required: Gloves—to prevent cuts, abrasions, and punctures?				
Metal-toed safety shoes, or at least strap-on metal foot shields—to prevent foot injuries?				
Receiving and Waste Disposal Areas Are crates, cartons, etc., opened away from open food containers?				
Are floors and docks cleared of refuse on a regular schedule (collection at least two, preferably three, times weekly)?				
Are garbage cans washed daily in hot water?				

Source: Adapted, with permission, from National Safety Council. *Long Term Care Safety Management Manual: A Handbook for Practical Application.* Chicago: National Safety Council, 1987, pp. 135–65.

Item	Yes	No	Comments on Deficiencies Noted and Action Required	Date Corrected
Are garbage cans always kept covered?				
Are garbage cans leakproof and adequate in number and size?				
Are garbage containers on dollies secured to racks?				
Are mops hung up where air can circulate?				
Are storage racks provided for cleaning equipment and is their use enforced (no equipment merely leaning against the walls)?				
Are oily rags kept in closed metal containers?				
Storage Areas—General Is storage space adequate to give everything a place and prevent "temporary" storage in the receiving area or hallways?				
Is it large enough to give employees room to bend their knees to lift?				
Is storage space provided for equipment, utensils, and supplies needed in work areas?				
Is shelving adequate to bear the weight of items stored?				
Is each employee instructed to store heavy items on lower shelves and lighter materials above?				
Is shelving adequately spaced to prevent pinching of hands?				
Are there enough portable and stationary storage racks in safe condition (free from broken or bent shelves and set on solid legs)?				

Source: Adapted, with permission, from National Safety Council. *Long Term Care Safety Management Manual: A Handbook for Practical Application.* Chicago: National Safety Council, 1987, pp. 135–65.

Item	Yes	No	Comments on Deficiencies Noted and Action Required	Date Corrected
Are all employees taught how to place their hands in order to move portable racks without injuring their hands?				
Are employees instructed not to store coats and other personal items in the storage room?				
Dry Storage Areas (*storeroom or kitchen*) Do cupboards have sliding doors?				
If not, are doors kept shut?				
Is storage of foodstuffs completely separate from storage of cleaning powders, insecticides, and other poisonous substances?				
Is a safe ladder provided for reaching high storage?				
Are flammable items kept at least 2 feet from light bulbs?				
Are light bulbs provided with screen guards?				
Cold Storage Areas (*walk-in and reach-in refrigerators*) Are the size of the refrigerator and the placement of the shelves such that all foods requiring refrigeration can be placed directly on shelves and in bins (rather than stacked one item on another)?				
Is the refrigerator located so that its door does not swing into and block a major traffic-way or corridor when opened?				
Is care taken to avoid breakage of food containers: Are nonbreakable types (plastic or metal) used when possible?				

Source: Adapted, with permission, from National Safety Council. *Long Term Care Safety Management Manual: A Handbook for Practical Application*. Chicago: National Safety Council, 1987, pp. 135–65.

Item	Yes	No	Comments on Deficiencies Noted and Action Required	Date Corrected
Are "flame- and oven-proof" glass and ceramic containers of food not moved directly from refrigerator to burner or preheated oven; from range or oven to refrigerator?				
Are thermostats kept in the refrigerators to provide easy checking for proper temperature?				
In walk-in refrigerators, is a device installed to permit emergency exit, either a bypass device on the door or an alarm bell?				
In walk-in refrigerators, is a screen or mesh guard provided around every blower fan?				
Food Preparation Areas *Cooking Area* Are employees using ranges, ovens, and broilers given the following basic instructions: On gas types, keep the burners clean and the gas and air intake properly adjusted.				
Dust behind and under the range weekly.				
Never allow grease to collect in cracks or on trays.				
Clean grease filters and range exhaust hoods at least once a week.				
Do not have curtains near flames or hot electric burners.				
Keep utensil handles turned away from the front of the stove, burners, and pilot lights.				
Use only dry pot holders. Keep them away from burners and pilot lights, and request new ones when needed.				

Source: Adapted, with permission, from National Safety Council. *Long Term Care Safety Management Manual: A Handbook for Practical Application.* Chicago: National Safety Council, 1987, pp. 135–65.

From *Safety Guide for Healthcare Institutions*, 4th edition, published by American Hospital Publishing, copyright 1989.

Item	Yes	No	Comments on Deficiencies Noted and Action Required	Date Corrected
Keep stove hoods clean and replace filters when dirty.				
To observe a cooking item, lift the side of the lid away from you to prevent steam burns.				
Avoid boil-overs by using a minimum amount of liquid and heat.				
Have a dry chemical or carbon dioxide fire extinguisher handy—and know how to use it.				
If a fire occurs in a cooking vessel, try to smother it with its lid or use a dry chemical or carbon dioxide fire extinguisher. Do not use water, flour, or other materials to extinguish grease fires.				
Stand to one side to light a gas oven. Before closing the oven door, always check to be sure the gas is ignited.				
Do not use cracked ceramic broiler burners; report or replace them.				
Remove grease drippings from the broiler after each use.				
Serving Area In that portion of the food preparation area where food is dished up or set out for pickup and service, are the following precautions observed: Is counter space provided between the stove and the dining room entrance so that attendants can pick up hot food without going near the stove?				
Is the employee handling hot packs or batteries for vacuum-sealed meal servers provided with gloves?				
Is counter space provided for setting out servings of cold food for pickup in the vicinity of either the refrigerator or the dining room entrance?				

Source: Adapted, with permission, from National Safety Council. *Long Term Care Safety Management Manual: A Handbook for Practical Application.* Chicago: National Safety Council, 1987, pp. 135–65.

Item	Yes	No	Comments on Deficiencies Noted and Action Required	Date Corrected
Is each employee carrying food to the dining room taught how to load—heaviest object in the center and cold food picked up before hot food?				
Is the traffic flow planned so that attendants do not collide while obtaining foods or carrying trays into the dining area?				
Is there glass in the door between the serving area and the dining room so that employees can see one another's approach?				
Is each side of swinging door marked IN or OUT to indicate its use?				
If necessary, are doors between the serving area and the dining area prevented from swinging into a dining room traffic area by a waist-high rail backstop that restricts door opening to 90 degrees and prevents persons from walking into the door?				
If carts are used to transport food to the dining room: Is traffic-free storage space provided for them in the serving area?				
Are they fitted to hold the food containers securely?				
Are employees trained in proper procedures for their use?				
Meal Service Areas: Dining Room—Long-Term Care Facilities Is the dining area itself safely arranged and maintained in safe condition: Are drapes, blinds, and curtains of fire-resistant materials?				
Are pictures and drapes securely fastened to walls?				

Source: Adapted, with permission, from National Safety Council. *Long Term Care Safety Management Manual: A Handbook for Practical Application.* Chicago: National Safety Council, 1987, pp. 135–65.

From *Safety Guide for Healthcare Institutions*, 4th edition, published by American Hospital Publishing, copyright 1989.

Item	Yes	No	Comments on Deficiencies Noted and Action Required	Date Corrected
Are chairs inspected weekly for splinters, metal burrs, and broken or loose parts, and removed for repair if defective?				
Are tables placed to allow aisle space for removal of dishes without lifting trays or food over the heads of diners?				
Are bus trucks or racks used to remove soiled dishes kept in safe condition (all wheels or casters working, all shelves firm)?				
Are there special provisions for serving "messy eaters" to facilitate cleanup and reduce fall hazards (separate section, ready availability of cleaning equipment and personnel)?				
Are separate ashtrays provided for all smokers?				
Are ashtrays emptied into metal containers?				
Are the activities of patients in the dining area supervised so that: They do not congregate at the dining room entrance prior to mealtime (to prevent falls caused by pushing or due to fatigue from standing in line).				
They receive assistance, if needed, in sitting down or rising from the table.				
Those who will not sit quietly are kept from wandering about the dining room and getting in the way of the attendants who are serving and clearing the tables (they are either escorted from the dining room or mildly restrained by use of a chair with a tray table).				
Those who are inclined to slide down in their chairs are provided with support, such as a chair with a tray table and a crotch strap.				

Source: Adapted, with permission, from National Safety Council. *Long Term Care Safety Management Manual: A Handbook for Practical Application.* Chicago: National Safety Council, 1987, pp. 135–65.

Item	Yes	No	Comments on Deficiencies Noted and Action Required	Date Corrected
Are attendants instructed in the serving and clearing procedures necessary to prevent injury to patients and themselves?				
Does the supervisor see that they follow these procedures: Attendants must always be ready to prevent an accident, for patients may make unexpected, nonrational moves.				
Attendants must announce their presence by saying "safety" or another generally agreed-upon warning when approaching one another, and particularly when passing behind patients and fellow attendants.				
Attendants guard against burns from spilled hot beverages by: Always pouring hot liquids for patients.				
Pouring a hot beverage into a cup placed on the table at the patient's right (not into a cup away from the table and passing the cup in front of the patient or over his or her head).				
Keeping group-sized pots or pitchers on a serving stand (not on tables) so that patients will not attempt to serve themselves.				
Removing spillage and breakage immediately, placing a chair over the hazardous area and having another attendant "guard" it while they are getting the cleaning equipment.				
When clearing tables, loading trays with heavy items in the center, china and glassware separated, and glasses not nested.				

Source: Adapted, with permission, from National Safety Council. *Long Term Care Safety Management Manual: A Handbook for Practical Application*. Chicago: National Safety Council, 1987, pp. 135–65.

Item	Yes	No	Comments on Deficiencies Noted and Action Required	Date Corrected
Room Tray Service Is the food (wherever possible) transported from the serving area to the patient's room on a cart rather than carried by hand on a tray?				
Does one attendant watch the food cart while another takes the tray into the patient's room in order to prevent possible injury to ambulatory residents who might come in contact with hot items on the cart?				
Is a table available in the room to place the tray on? (The tray should not be balanced on a pillow or the knees, or placed on a mattress.)				
Is the attendant serving meals in rooms trained in the following safe practices: Make space for the tray in the room before bringing the tray into the room.				
Do not overload the tray or the cart, and put liquids toward the center.				
Keep food covered when in transit.				
Do not block corridors or doorways with the cart.				
Keep the wheels in line with the cart to prevent a tripping hazard.				
Avoid spillage by not overloading trays, bowls, or cups; clean up spillage at once.				
Remove the tray as soon as the patient has finished the meal.				
Serve no foods that during transit have been subjected to unsanitary handling or exposed to broken glass or crockery.				

Source: Adapted, with permission, from National Safety Council. *Long Term Care Safety Management Manual: A Handbook for Practical Application.* Chicago: National Safety Council, 1987, pp. 135–65.

Item	Yes	No	Comments on Deficiencies Noted and Action Required	Date Corrected
Washing Areas Are racks in safe condition (if wooden, free of broken slats and splinters; if metal, free of sharp corners that could cause cuts)?				
Are racks kept off the floor to prevent tripping hazards?				
Are drainboards large enough for draining without pyramid stacking?				
Are drain plugs of the type that permit draining without an employee reaching his or her hand down into the water?				
Are adequate rubber gloves provided?				
Is a thermometer used to determine that water temperatures are safe?				
Are employees instructed not to use sharp-edged cans as utensils?				
Are employees instructed as to the correct amounts of detergent and other cleaning agents to be used?				
Are employees given the following special instructions for handling glassware (in addition to the general instructions): Do not crowd racks or conveyors when racking dishes or glassware.				
Do not tilt glassware in the washer.				
Do not mix china, silver, and glassware in the same rack.				
Do not place or wash dishes and glasses in a pot-washing sink.				
Drain dish tanks to remove broken china and glassware.				

Source: Adapted, with permission, from National Safety Council. *Long Term Care Safety Management Manual: A Handbook for Practical Application.* Chicago: National Safety Council, 1987, pp. 135–65.

From *Safety Guide for Healthcare Institutions*, 4th edition, published by American Hospital Publishing, copyright 1989.

Item	Yes	No	Comments on Deficiencies Noted and Action Required	Date Corrected
General Are food cart wheels and drawers in good repair?				
Are all gauges in good working order?				
Are dumbwaiters securely shut when not in use?				
Are steam, gas, and water pipes clearly marked for identification?				
Are knives kept sharpened and in good condition?				
Are cuts always made away from the body?				
Are knives, saws, and cleavers kept in designated areas when not in use?				
Are blades stored with the cutting edge covered?				
Is hand protection readily available for handling hot utensils?				
Do employees stand to the side of a unit when lighting gas stoves and ovens?				
Are all exits, passageways, fire extinguishers, or electrical breaker panels clear of carts, boxes, trash cans, or other items?				
Are microwave ovens cleaned often?				
Are the door seals on the microwave ovens in good condition so that the door closes securely?				
Are heavy lids on equipment such as a steam kettle secured to prevent accidental falling?				
Do machines for slicing, grinding, cutting, etc., have guards on all toggle switches to prevent accidental starting?				

Source: Adapted, with permission, from National Safety Council. *Long Term Care Safety Management Manual: A Handbook for Practical Application.* Chicago: National Safety Council, 1987, pp. 135–65.

From *Safety Guide for Healthcare Institutions*, 4th edition, published by American Hospital Publishing, copyright 1989.

Item	**Yes**	**No**	**Comments on Deficiencies Noted and Action Required**	**Date Corrected**
Do walk-in freezers have an inside light switch and a means of opening the door from the inside?				
Are foodstuffs checked for foul smells, decomposed products, improperly maintained frozen/refrigerated foods, insect/rodent filth, and damaged/open cartons and bent cans?				
Are items stored on pallets or shelves to provide for floor cleaning?				
Is displayed food properly protected from contamination by display cases or other means, and maintained at the required temperature?				
Are ice machines clean, free of rust, and not used for food storage?				
Is ice stored in approved, closed containers?				
Are scoops used for ice stored in a holder outside the machine?				

Source: Adapted, with permission, from National Safety Council. *Long Term Care Safety Management Manual: A Handbook for Practical Application*. Chicago: National Safety Council, 1987, pp. 135–65.

From *Safety Guide for Healthcare Institutions, 4th edition, published by American Hospital Publishing, copyright 1989.*

Bibliography

Barton, E. L. Administration of psychotropic agents to patients who refuse such medication. *Perspectives in Healthcare Risk Management (ASHRM)* 8(4):13–14, Fall 1988.

Beatty, G. C. *Developing a Hospital Emergency Preparedness Program.* Chicago: American Society for Hospital Engineering, 1987.

Calandra, P. R. Simultaneous disasters result in greater hospital preparedness. *Perspectives in Healthcare Risk Management (ASHRM)* 7(4):13–14, Fall 1987.

Department of Labor and Department of Health and Human Services. *Protection Against Occupational Exposure to Hepatitis B Virus (HBV) and Human Immunodeficiency Virus (HIV). Joint Advisory Notice.* Washington, DC: DOL/HHS, Oct. 19, 1987.

Environmental Protection Agency. *Asbestos Waste Management Guidance.* Washington, DC: EPA, May 1985.

Environmental Protection Agency. *EPA Guide for Infectious Waste Management.* Washington, DC: EPA, May 1986.

Environmental Protection Agency. *Guidance for Controlling Asbestos-Containing Materials in Buildings.* Washington, DC: EPA, June 1985.

Environmental Protection Agency. *Understanding the Small Quantity Generator Hazardous Waste Rules: A Handbook for Small Business.* Washington, DC: EPA, Sept. 1986.

Feldman, R. H. L. Hospital injuries. *Occupational Health and Safety* 55(9):12–15, Sept. 1986.

Gagnon, M., Sicard, C., and Sirois, J. P. Evaluation of forces on the lumbo-sacral joint and assessment of work and energy transfers in nursing aides lifting patients. *Ergonomics* 29(3):407–21, Mar. 1986.

Gates, W. E. Mitigation of earthquake effects on hospital facilities. *Perspectives in Healthcare Risk Management (ASHRM)* 7(4):15–21, Fall 1987.

Joint Commission on Accreditation of Healthcare Organizations. *The KIPS Survey Guide for 1989: Hospital Accreditation Program.* Chicago: JCAHO, 1988.

Joseph, E. D. Strengthening risk management in psychiatric facilities. *Perspectives in Healthcare Risk Management (ASHRM)* 8(4):15–18, Fall 1988.

Leska, M. Preparing a hospital's nuclear disaster plan. *Perspectives in Healthcare Risk Management (ASHRM)* 7(4):11–12, Fall 1987.

Magazine, C. J. Investigating staff abuse of patients in psychiatric setting. *Perspectives in Healthcare Risk Management (ASHRM)* 8(4):19–22, Fall 1988.

McCormick, R. D., and Maki, D. G. Epidemiology of needle-stick injuries in hospital personnel. *American Journal of Medicine* 9(4):928–32, Apr. 1981.

Morgan, V., and others. Hospital falls: a persistent problem. *American Journal of Public Health* 75(7):775–77, July 1985.

National Fire Protection Association. *Health Care Safety Reports and Articles.* Quincy, MA: NFPA, 1987.

Occupational Safety and Health Administration. Instruction CPL 2-2.44A. *Enforcement Procedures for Occupational Exposure to Hepatitis B Virus (HBV) and Human Immunodeficiency Virus (HIV).* Washington, DC: OSHA, Aug. 15, 1988.

Occupational Safety and Health Administration. Instruction PUB 8-1.1. *Work Practice Guidelines for Personnel Dealing with Cytotoxic (Antineoplastic) Drugs.* Washington, DC: OSHA, Jan. 29, 1986.

O'Mara, S. C. Earthquake survey reveals need for focused hospital disaster planning. *Perspectives in Healthcare Risk Management (ASHRM)* 8(2):24–25, Spring 1988.

Orlikoff, J. E., and Vanagunas, A. M. *Malpractice Prevention and Liability Control for Hospitals.* 2nd ed. Chicago: American Hospital Publishing, 1988.

Rusting, R. Special report: patient falls update—new approaches. *Hospital Security and Safety Management* 6(7):5–8, Nov. 1985.

Rusting, R., and Nelson, V. Successful patient restraint while avoiding abuse. *Nursing Home Security and Safety Management* 2(9):2–4, May 1984.

Slavik, N. S. *Hazardous Waste Management Strategies for Health Care Facilities.* Chicago: American Hospital Association, 1987.

Sorock, G. S. A case control study of falling incidents among the hospitalized elderly. *Journal of Safety Research* 14(2):47–52, Summer 1983.

Tan, M. W. Suicide and violence to others: loss prevention strategies. *Perspectives in Healthcare Risk Management (ASHRM)* 8(4):9–12, Fall 1988.

Wade, R. D. *Risk Management—HPL, Hospital Professional Liability Primer.* Columbus, OH: Ohio Insurance Company, 1983.

Index